Acknowledgments

We would like to thank the following individuals for their generous contribution of time, expertise, and moral support in the production of this monograph:

Henriette Davis
Sandra Fraser
Greg Hendrick
Shirley Hendrick
Karen Luxton
Amy Underhill
Myrna Vota
Sarah Barbara Watstein
David Wilkinson
John Wilkinson
Diane Wolfe

We would like to extend a very special thank you to Ann Hope, LITA Monograph Series Editor.

Chapter One

Introduction

While the ability to record information permanently by means of a linear code has contributed immeasurably to humankind's intellectual progress, the development of the earliest writing system was regarded with disdain by the ancient Greeks. In the *Phaedrus*, Plato describes Socrates' scornful reaction to the invention of writing: "Those who use writing will become forgetful, relying on an external resource for what they lack in internal resources."[1] Indeed, the end of the oral tradition signaled not only the potential deterioration of the human memory but also the beginning of our reliance upon sight to process information.

We are, as a civilization, dominated by our visual perception. As librarians we can hardly conceive of information being stored and transmitted in any form other than print. Certainly, technological advances made in recent decades have familiarized us all with so-called machine-readable formats, but generally we think of information as existing in some form of print. How, then, are the blind or visually impaired to obtain this information which, by its very nature, seems unavailable to them? This book attempts to outline the diverse ways in which information can be made accessible to individuals for whom print is a seemingly exclusionary medium.

Most of us assume that the primary method of information exchange available to the blind and visually impaired is braille, the well-known system of raised dot configurations which transcribes the orthography and syntax of the language in question. While braille is still commonly used by many visually impaired individuals, it can no longer be considered the primary method of information exchange despite the fact that for many print-impaired people it is still the most efficient means of storing information in true written format. Taking notes in the classroom, writing down phone numbers or grocery lists, and labeling cans in the pantry are all tasks that are frequently best performed with a braille writing device. However, such things as bank statements, telephone directories, and library card catalogs are not generally produced in braille; those who are print impaired must find alternative means to access the vast majority of information that is available in our society.

It should be noted that knowledge of braille is generally limited to the blind and visually impaired, sometimes extending to their families, friends, and rehabilitation counselors. The general population is not braille literate, nor can we expect that it might become so. Thus, as with members of the hearing-impaired community who have, by necessity, learned to lip-read and/or speak, the print-impaired individual must find another route than braille for information exchange with the sighted population. One such alternative is the use of audiocassettes and microcomputers equipped with adaptive devices such as screen-enlargers and/or synthetic speech programs. This is not to suggest that the use of audiocassettes or microcomputers should completely supplant the use of braille within the print-impaired community; rather, these media can be used together with older techniques to maximize the potential degree of access one has to varied types of information. Although the zipper is a newer technology than the button, it is unlikely that anyone within the garment industry would want it to replace the button completely: both methods of fastening clothes are in use today, each having its own application, and neither has been eliminated by the use of velcro—a newer technology still.

Thus, when we seek to make our programs and facilities available to the print-impaired patron, we must be aware of the many methodological options that now exist. We must understand the value of each and plan accordingly. In the following chapters, we hope to increase the reader's awareness of the variety of systems available and the advantages and disadvantages of each. We have taken into account factors such as budgetary constraints, spacial restrictions, and staffing limitations. Ultimately, our goal has been to help unravel the paradox of how best to integrate the print-impaired individual into an environment where integration depends so profoundly on access to print documents.

Although we have taken somewhat of a historical approach to our discussion of access systems, chapter 2 begins with an introduction to computer terminology and then proceeds to an overview of some of the newest technological advances to have benefitted our target population. Here we explore not only the ubiquitous presence of the microcomputer but also several devices ("stand-alones" and "peripherals") whose development and subsequent proliferation has been largely due to cost reductions resulting from the mass-production of microcomputer technology. In this section, we will discuss optical character recognition, telecommunications, and local area networks. Included is an examination of trends, such as the growing use of the graphical user interface (GUI), that may be perceived as problematic to the visually impaired user. The purpose of this chapter is to situate our readers within the context of the most recent advances so that they may better evaluate the progress that has been made since Valentin Haüy opened his school for the blind in Paris over two hundred years ago.

Chapter 3 focuses on the use of braille and other tactile access systems. The development of the earliest touch-oriented writing codes is traced. We explain the fundamentals of Louis Braille's enduring system and discuss the reasons for its longevity. Each of the electronic devices (such as braille embossers and soft-braille systems) that has helped to incorporate the use of braille in the technological age is described. Acquisition of braille texts is explored through a detailed discussion of the National Library Service for the Blind and Physically Handicapped (NLS) as well as other agencies that produce hundreds of new braille titles annually. Since new technologies have rendered the production of braille relatively inexpensive and virtually as simple as standard word processing, this section also includes an examination of in-house production of braille materials.

Where chapter 3 is primarily concerned with the use of tactile access systems, chapter 4 outlines the development of auditory-based media, beginning with Thomas Edison's inclusion of "recorded books for blind people" in his 1877 patent on the phonograph.[2] The production and dissemination of recorded materials by agencies such as the NLS and Recording for the Blind (RFB) is described with a focus on copyright agreements and eligibility requirements. Much of the chapter is devoted to an examination of adaptive technologies that enable the blind or visually impaired individual to interact with computer systems via synthetic speech output. A variety of screen-access systems are briefly reviewed and the reader is supplied with a set of selection criteria and purchasing guidelines. Issues related to training for both library staff and individual end users are addressed. Again, processes relating to both the acquisition and production of machine-readable texts are described. Although the development of adaptive hardware and software has done much to promote the academic and socioeconomic independence of the disabled community as a whole, recent technological trends (e.g., the graphical user interface mentioned earlier) pose a formidable threat to this independence. The reasons why the GUIs are incompatible with the design of current screen-access systems are explained and the reader is provided with a survey of current research into the problem.

Chapter 5 is predominantly concerned with the ways in which individuals having low vision may be accommodated. Since terms such as "partially sighted" and "legally blind" tend to encompass a broad range of individuals with varying degrees of vision loss, we open this chapter with a series of useful definitions including those used by various state agencies, private institutions, and library services serving the blind and visually impaired. Given the potential disparity among individuals categorized as having low vision, the range of so-called adaptive devices discussed in this section is quite broad. From conventional magnifying glasses to sophisticated computer screen-enhancement hard- and software, the production of large print materials is described in detail. As most modern libraries are now equipped with standard laser printers that can generate high-quality text as large as 24 point and beyond, some attention is directed toward examination of off-the-shelf software that can be used to produce accessible text formats. Guidelines for using diverse fonts (styles, sizes, and attributes) are presented.

Accommodating the print-impaired patron entails much more than providing access to the collection of books and periodicals itself. He or she must be able to search the card catalog independently, retrieve materials from the stacks with limited assistance, and be informed of and able to participate in each of the activities offered to the sighted patron. Chapter 6 discusses access to a variety of standard programs and services. Suggestions regarding acquisitions, training, and community outreach are offered. In two separate sections, we outline specifications for the creation of a library access center. There is a description of the ideal configuration, where few budgetary constraints apply, as well as a proposal for those working within a moderate budget.

The Print-Impaired Reader

Before exploring the range of services and types of materials available for print-impaired readers, we must consider the population we are serving, and clarify some of the definitions of this seemingly jargon-ridden field. We use the expression "print-impaired" to describe any literate person who cannot independently read the printed page, exclusive of people with physical or mobility-related disabilities. Therefore, the needs of people who cannot comfortably hold a book, or turn its pages, for example, will not be addressed here. Included in our use of "print-impaired" are readers with varying degrees of vision loss, from the totally blind reader to the occasional user of a magnifying glass for very fine print.

Also included in our use of the term "print-impaired" are people with learning disabilities, many of whom can benefit from some of the same reading aids used by people with visual impairments. People with learning disabilities exhibit difficulties in processing information. Unlike the visually impaired reader, who has difficulty seeing print, the learning disabled reader can see but may not process print as effectively as others, that is, has difficulty with certain cognitive processes associated with reading. At the turn of the century, acknowledgement of the existence of learning disabilities came from baffled physicians whose patients could not read although vision, speech, and intelligence remained intact. They referred to this condition as "word blindness."

It wasn't until the 1920s that physicians came to question some of our assumptions about learning and learning difficulties. In 1925, Dr. Samuel T. Orton, a neurologist and psychiatrist at the Iowa Psychopathic Hospital, proposed the existence of a physical basis for reading problems that went against the prevailing belief that learning difficulties were the result of emotional problems.[3] We now know that some learning problems are indeed physically based, but research has shown that learners afflicted with physically based learning disabilities can be taught strategies to compensate for their disability.

Although significant progress has been made in the areas of diagnosis and remedial education of people with learning disabilities, there is still no single, universally accepted definition of this class of disabilities. The most commonly used definition of "learning-disabled" can be found in PL 94-142, The Education of All Handicapped Children Act of 1975:

> The term "children with specific learning disabilities" means those children who have a disorder in one or more of the basic psychological processes involved in understanding or in using language, spoken or written, which disorder may manifest itself in imperfect ability to listen, think, speak, read, write, spell, or do mathematical calculations. Such disorders include such conditions as perceptual handicaps, brain injury, minimal brain dysfunction, dyslexia, and developmental aphasia. Such term does not include children who have learning problems which are primarily the result of visual, hearing, or motor handicaps; of mental retardation; of emotional disturbance; or of environmental, cultural or economic disadvantage.

PL 94-142 had far-reaching consequences for not only the learning disabled, but also for school-age children with other disabilities. The ultimate effect of PL 94-142 was to assure access to a free public education, with reasonable accommodations made for the student's effective participation in instructional programs.

In practical terms, the learning disability might manifest itself as a very slow reading speed, as slow as three to four pages of print per hour. An inability to comprehend and effectively use many of the library's basic tools, such as card catalogs and periodical indexes, also characterizes many learning-disabled library patrons. Difficulty with concepts like the alphanumeric arrangement of Library of Congress call numbers, for example, can make using the library intensely frustrating for some people with learning disabilities. Often, and unfortunately, the learning-disabled reader will just give up. Admitting to being unable to deal with what seem like very simple tasks can be extremely difficult; consequently, many learning-disabled people remain "in the closet" about their disability.

Librarians with an understanding of learning disabilities can provide a much needed service to this segment of the library's user population. In our discussion of audio-based reading aids (chapter 4), we will consider sources of alternative materials for this often overlooked segment of the library's clientele.

Accessible Texts

Our use of the term "accessible text" refers to any or all of the following adaptations of print materials: sound recordings in the form of cassette tapes or audio records, braille or other embossed texts, electronic texts (used primarily with computer-based synthetic speech programs), or large print materials. Further clarification is required for emerging electronic information media. CD-ROM products, for example, are accessible texts (ROM means "read-only memory"), even though few libraries presently own the synthetic speech or large print technology required for independent access to them by print-impaired individuals. Similarly, online sources such as Dialog, RLIN (Research Libraries Information Network), or the local online public access catalog (OPAC) are accessible, but only with the use of "adaptive technology."

"Adaptive technology," another term bandied about since the introduction of the personal computer in the 1980s, refers to any software or hardware addition to the computer that renders it accessible to a person with special needs. Included are large print computer displays, synthetic speech programs that read aloud the contents of the computer screen, etc.

We should also define two terms that we use throughout the monograph and that many of us probably take for granted. We all think we know what "reading" means. One of the dictionary definitions for the verb "to read" is "to have the knowledge of (a language) necessary to understand printed or written material."[4] Our definition of reading encompasses more than the simple decoding of printed materials; for our purposes, the reader who listens to *Wuthering Heights* on tape is "reading" *Wuthering Heights*. Similarly, we should bear in mind that we read for many different reasons, and in different ways. Our leisurely reading of a mystery novel for entertainment, for example, differs from the way we study a textbook, which in turn differs from the way we consult a telephone book. For the print-impaired reader, different types of reading may lend themselves to different media. Given the full spectrum of choices, for example, few blind readers would choose to listen to a novel with synthetic speech; rather, they will probably opt for an audio recording of the text. Similarly, few computer-literate visually impaired readers would select an audio tape dictionary over a machine-readable one. Using the power of a computer equipped with synthetic speech, the reader can pinpoint a dictionary entry almost instantly; imagine trying to use the tape recorder's "fast forward" button to locate a single word?

Our responsibility to disseminate information and provide access to a diverse collection of written documents extends to all members of the population. The shelves of our libraries are stocked with works as philosophically, stylistically, and linguistically varied as the patrons we serve. When we have an opportunity to improve service to a particular contingent of the population, we should seize it. Now that technology has provided us with new means to aid the print impaired, we are obliged to act. The following chapters are designed to assist in that process.

Notes

1. Walter Ong, *Orality and Literacy* (New York: Methuen, 1982), 79.
2. "A History of the National Library Service for Blind and Physically Handicapped Individuals, The Library of Congress" in *That All May Read* (Washington, D.C.: Library of Congress, 1983), 80.
3. Barbara Bliss, "Dyslexics as Library Users," *Library Trends* 35 (Fall 1986): 294.
4. *American Heritage Dictionary of the English Language*, s.v. "read."

Chapter Two

A Crash Course
in Computer Literacy

Virtually any discussion of access to print for blind, visually impaired, and learning-disabled readers will inevitably turn to an examination of microprocessing technology, for it is primarily through the use of computers that our target population will be fully integrated into the mainstream library environment. While media such as braille, large print, and the audiocassette were commonly in use among print-impaired readers prior to the introduction of the personal computer, reliance upon special text formats cannot empower this community in the same way or to the same extent as does the ability to access standard materials and equipment by means of adaptive technology. Computerized card catalogs, online database systems, electronic mail, and word processors have all contributed immeasurably to the general public's professional and academic productivity; the use of these same technologies has revolutionized accessibility for print-impaired individuals.

Text files stored on computer disk are easily read by the blind or visually impaired user with the help of a synthetic speech device, refreshable braille system, or screen-enlarging software package. Papers and reports are just as easily modified and manipulated within standard word processors using any number of adaptive technologies. Braille embossers and laser printers enable the production of hard copy in accessible formats. Even print materials are rendered accessible through the use of optical character recognition devices. Chapters 3, 4, and 5 are devoted to explicit discussions of the nature and variety of the adaptive products available for use by blind, visually impaired, and learning-disabled computer users, but these sections assume some degree of computer literacy. For the reader who is less than a computerphile, these discussions may prove confusing. In the following pages, we offer definitions of many of the terms used throughout the text and attempt to unlock the mystery of several important concepts involved in microprocessing technology.

The Microcomputer

Although the term *PC* has come to be used interchangeably with *desktop* or *home computer*, it was originally a product name coined by IBM when the company introduced its first commercially viable microcomputer in 1981. However, like *Xerox* and *Kleenex*, the term *PC*, which is, of course, an abbreviation for personal computer, has now acquired generic noun status. Today, all personal computers that are IBM compatible are considered PCs. Indeed, the reader will shortly discover that the term PC is used throughout this monograph as a synonym for personal, desktop, or home computer. On the other hand, Apple computers are not generally referred to as PCs though they are microcomputers.

Hardware and Software

Modern PCs, called fourth-generation computers, rely upon silicon chips to perform a variety of computational tasks. These tiny silicon flakes are actually integrated circuits which have the advantage of being small, inexpensive, and fast. The rate at which they process information is measured in MIPS or million instructions per second. Perhaps the most important of all the chips found inside any microcomputer is the central processing unit or CPU. The CPU is the computer's commander-in-chief, responsible for all aspects of data processing. When we refer to a computer as an *8088*, *286*, or *386*, we are referring to the model number of the CPU. Despite standard nomenclature, the CPU is not, however, the big box on which most users place their monitors; rather, it is one of the chips found on the mother board inside the case.

The computer case, with all the essential innerworkings, is called the system unit. The system unit is, of course, where all processing takes place, but it is not technically called the CPU. Indeed, the system unit contains far more than this one chip: the mother board, floppy drives, hard disk, controller cards, power supply, expansion boards, etc. All input and output devices and external peripherals are attached to the system unit. It is one of the computer's three main hardware components. The other two main hardware components are the system keyboard and the monitor. The keyboard is an input device since the operator uses this mechanism to enter data. Light pens, mice, and voice recognition systems are all examples of input devices. The monitor is an output device, so named because it is the device through which data are conveyed to the user. Printers and synthetic speech devices are also considered output systems.

Hardware, then, refers to any physical piece of computer equipment that may be handled—the actual nuts and bolts of the system. Conversely, software is intangible; while computer programs and data may be stored on physical disks, the actual instructions that comprise the program are not really material objects. Firmware is a combination of hard- and software. For example, the ROM BIOS, crucial information stored on a computer chip, is called firmware.

Memory and Storage Capacity

Any discussion of tangible versus intangible within the context of micro-computers must include an explanation of the difference between memory and storage capacity. Often new users will confuse these two concepts, but in fact they are distinct entities. Perhaps the only similarity between memory and storage capacity lies in the unit of measurement used to register size. Computers measure information in units called bytes, which are made up of smaller units called bits. Bit is an abbreviation for *binary digit*, since these units are based on a binary code having but two significant numbers: 0 and 1. These zeros and ones correspond, respectively, to the off and on state of a circuit. It is through this series of continuous offs and ons that the computer transmits data. Of course, any number could be repre-sented in binary code, given enough digits. However, each byte consists of but eight binary digits or bits so that this code can only represent the numbers 0 through 255. ASCII (the American Standard Code for Informa-tion Interchange) was developed in 1965 to facilitate the binary represen-tation of all the characters one might enter from a computer keyboard. The standard ASCII character set consists of 128 numbers ranging from 0 to 127. These numbers are assigned to letters, numbers, punctuation marks, and a variety of special characters. The extended ASCII character set ranges from 128 to 255, and is assigned to foreign characters, mathematical symbols, and graphics. For example, when the user strikes the "a" key on the keyboard, an ASCII 97 is issued which, in turn, corresponds to a series of eight binary digits set to 0 or 1. Each time a key is struck, the computer recognizes one byte of information—turning its circuits on and off in exact correlation with the configuration of 1s and 0s used to express that number.

The number of bytes the computer can address at any one time deter-mines its memory capacity; that is, just how much data the system can "retain" in its "mind" at any given moment. As might be expected, the capacity of computer disks, which are magnetic storage media, is also calculated in terms of bytes, but the amount of information that can be stored on a disk and the amount of information the computer can address at a given moment are grossly inequivalent. Consider an analogy between the brain and a microprocessor: The human mind is able to store far more information than it can process simultaneously. We may know how to multiply, speak a foreign language, play the piano, and bake a cake, but we are not able to perform all of these tasks at once. Our individual memory capacities will fill up after just a few "commands" are executed: MULTI-PLY.EXE, SPEAKFORN.EXE may be the best we can do before our "random access memory" is depleted. And yet, we still store the instruction set for PIANO.EXE and BAKECAKE.EXE and as soon as we stop multiplying and speaking the foreign language we may commence one of these other activities. We will have freed up enough room in our mental faculty to undertake a different task. The computer operates in much the same manner. Its memory capacity is fixed and the number of tasks it can accomplish at any one time is dependent upon the limitation of just how much data must be read from each individual instruction set.

Now let us expand our analogy to illustrate the difference between RAM (random-access memory) and ROM (read-only memory). While we are multiplying and speaking the foreign language, we do not forget to breathe or circulate blood through our veins or have our heart beat. The instruction set for these crucial activities is stored and carried out somewhere outside the part of our brain that tells us how to speak and perform mathematical operations. The mechanisms that cause us to breathe, pump blood, and maintain a heartbeat are involuntary—they continue to operate even when we are asleep—"turned off," as it were. We cannot reallocate this portion of our brain for use by activities such as playing the piano, for not only would we fail to execute PIANO.EXE properly but our systems would shut down completely. The instructions stored in the computer's ROM are symbolic of its involuntary reflexes. ROM is stored on a separate chip and is inviolable; it does not shut down when the computer is "asleep"—turned off. ROM is preconfigured by the computer manufacturer. It is unalterable—hence the name "read-only"—and completely unerasable.

When we speak of a computer's memory capacity, however, we most generally make reference to the RAM since this is the type of memory that is of greatest interest to the individual user. Data associated with operating system files, applications programs, adaptive software, and information entered from the console will consume some degree of RAM. All microprocessors, beginning with Intel's 8088 chip, are capable of addressing 1,048,576 bytes of conventional memory. This figure is referred to as a megabyte (MB). In binary terms, "mega" is roughly equivalent to the decimal number million. One "meg" or 1,048,576 is the result of 2 raised to the twentieth power. A kilobyte (K), similar to the decimal number thousand, is 2 to the tenth power, or 1,024. DOS (the disk operating system), and its applications are designed to consume less than the first 640K of conventional memory. The remaining 394K is generally used by other aspects of the system such as the video RAM, machine bios, and the like. This upper memory area can, however, be exploited by software applications designed to use expanded and/or extended memory.

The difference between expanded (EMS) and extended (XMS) memory can be somewhat elusive. Both reside in the same upper memory area above the 640K barrier but the way in which the data are accessed and subsequently processed differs considerably from expanded to extended memory. All of Intel's CPU chips can take advantage of expanded memory but only the 80286, 80386, and 80486 chips can use extended memory. Since most adaptive programs are memory resident, meaning that they remain in memory until disabled by the user or until the system is powered down (turned off), those packages that can take advantage of the upper memory area are preferable to those that consume precious conventional memory. DOS 5, the newest version of Microsoft's product, can be loaded into the upper memory area as well, freeing more conventional memory for applications that are not generally designed to load "high," i.e., in the upper memory area.[1]

Let's reconsider our previous analogy: imagine that the human mind had a kind of upper memory area where the information required for performing one or another task could be processed, and that this memory area would not interfere with information being processed in other areas of the brain. Under these conditions, one probably could multiply a series of numbers, speak a foreign language, play the piano, and bake a cake all at once. Indeed, operating systems that can establish what is known as "protected mode" enable this type of multitasking. Multitasking, or the ability to run two or more applications at once, is not available under DOS but there are several operating systems that do support this feature, which may prove to be invaluable to the print-impaired user.

The Operating System

The computer's operating system is the master program under which all applications software run. Word processors, database systems, spreadsheets, telecommunications software, and adaptive devices must be compatible with the operating system in use in order to function properly. By and large, the most common operating system used by IBM and compatible computers today is DOS. PC-DOS was developed by Microsoft Corporation in the early 1980s to be used with the first of IBM's personal computers. In many regards, it was little more than a rewrite of an earlier operating system, CP/M, developed by Gary Kildall at Digital Research, Inc. (DRI). Later, when IBM clones began to infiltrate the computer market, Microsoft introduced MS-DOS, which is virtually identical to its predecessor. Microsoft's release of DOS version 5.0 in 1991 represented a considerable improvement over earlier versions in terms of memory management, system utilities, and documentation. However, even this newest version of the operating system does not enable multitasking, as briefly described in the previous section.

Most readers can surely imagine the advantages to an operating system that allows its users to run several applications at once; such extraordinary computational power can be of inestimable importance to the print-impaired user. Programs running in a multitasking environment are said to be in separate "windows"—prevented from interfering with one another by protective barriers set up by the operating system itself. The blind computer user whose system has multitasking capabilities can be composing a letter within a word processor, switch to another window to look up a needed name and address in a database file, switch back to the letter, add the name and address, and then switch to yet another window to extract financial information from a spreadsheet. All the while, this same user can be downloading files from a remote computer via a telecommunications package. Since many print-impaired computer users will have a greater dependency upon electronic information than sighted individuals who can simply glance through an ordinary Rolodex or checkbook, the independence of users whose systems are equipped with a substantial amount of memory, the ability to properly manage that memory, and to perform multitasking operations will be enormously increased.

Unfortunately, not all operating systems that support multitasking are equally speech-friendly because of their tendency to incorporate a graphical user interface (GUI). Indeed, systems such as OS/2, UNIX, and Microsoft Windows (which is actually designed to run under either DOS or OS/2) may prove problematic for a variety of adaptive technologies. The GUI, familiar to Macintosh users, relies upon an object-oriented screen display to render computer operation easier. Icons and other graphics images are used to convey information to the user, who often may select among them using some type of pointer, but this type of system is virtually inaccessible to the print-impaired individual who must rely upon speech or refreshable braille. In many cases, the GUI will be equally uninterpretable to screen-enlarging hardware products.[2]

The greatest advantage of DOS where the print-impaired user is concerned is, arguably, its so-called command line. Once a computer using MS-DOS as its operating system is booted up (turned on), the user may simply enter executable commands. These commands are issued as fairly logical text strings. For example, to obtain a listing of files in the current directory, the user would type DIR and then strike Enter. To change directories, the user types CHDIR or DIR, and the command to make a new directory is MKDIR or MD. Admittedly, this is not quite as elegant or nearly as much fun as clicking a mouse (the typical pointer in the GUI systems) on a picture of a file cabinet, disk, or some other mnemonic object, but for the print-impaired user who cannot easily navigate the video display with a mouse, using the keyboard to enter information on the command line is extremely user-friendly.

Fortunately, DESQview by Quarterdeck Office Systems, a powerful package used in conjunction with the company's QEMM (Quarterdeck Extended Memory Manager), provides print-impaired users with a happy solution to the problem. Not only does DESQview enable multitasking but, running under DOS, it retains the operating system's command line as well.

Computer Disks

Most of today's desktop computers are equipped with a hard or fixed disk on which the operating system, applications programs, and a variety of user files are stored, more or less permanently. Indeed, many of the features we have described in the preceding sections (memory management, multitasking, etc.) would be rendered virtually impossible without the benefits of a hard disk. In the absence of a hard disk, users have to store all operating system files, applications software, and data on individual floppy disks (sometimes called diskettes), changing them every time information that is not present on the current disk is needed. Running even moderately-sized programs results in constant disk switching. This was, of course, the nature of microcomputer operation in the early '80s before the hard disk was invented. Factor in the slowness of the original floppy drives and the low storage capacity of the disks themselves and the limitations of the pre-hard disk PC are mind-boggling by today's standards. One wonders how anyone could have regarded the original PC/XT class machines as anything but slightly more frustrating alternatives to fountain pens, index cards, and abacuses.

Floppy disks are magnetic storage media that come in two sizes: 5.25 inches and 3.5 inches in diameter. The larger disks are an older medium and hold less information than do the 3.5-inch disks, sometimes called microfloppies. In fact, the 3.5-inch microfloppies bear little resemblance to their 5.25-inch predecessors. Rigid in appearance because of a protective plastic case, the 3.5-inch disks are far less vulnerable to external damage than the 5.25-inch disks.

Although there are but two different sizes of floppy disks, both are available in either high- or low-density design. Whether or not a disk is a high-density disk is determined during the manufacturing process. High-density disks are coated with a special magnetic substance that allows more information to be stored on them. However, often the drives used to read from and write to the disks will dictate the amount of information that can be stored on each. Before a disk can be used, it must be formatted. This process, performed by an operating system command, prepares the disk for use by the computer. Formatting a disk accomplishes much the same task as drawing evenly spaced lines on blank notebook paper: not only is it much easier to write on paper that is ruled, but information written on this type of paper is far more easily read at a later date.

As we learned above, computer data, whether stored on a disk or present in memory, is always measured in terms of bytes, kilobytes, and megabytes. A low-density 5.25-inch drive will always format disks for 360K of storage capacity whether or not the disks are low-density disks. Similarly, a high-density 5.25-inch disk drive will format its disks high by default, whether or not these disks are truly high-density media. The high-density 5.25-inch drive nearly quadruples the storage capacity of a 5.25-inch disk from 360K to 1.2MB. It is important to note that a special command line parameter may be issued to cause the high-density drive to format a disk "low." In this way, disks formatted on a computer with a high-density drive may be read from and written to by a low-density drive. As might be expected, the high-density drives are capable of reading the 360K disks but the low-density drives are not able to read the 1.2MB disks. Unfortunately, the disk drives are identical in outward appearance so that users cannot tell whether a drive is high- or low-density just by looking at it. One reliable rule of thumb is that most PC and XT class machines are installed with low-density 5.25-inch drives while AT class computers will often have high-density drives.

In any case, it is inadvisable to format low-density disks high despite the fact that doing so augments the disk's storage capacity considerably. Formatting a low-density disk high generally results in the production of so-called "bad sectors," imperfections in the disk's storage system that can eventually lead to the destruction of data. Forcing a low-density disk to conform to a high format is much like forcing one's size 9 foot into a size 5 shoe—sooner or later there'll be trouble. Generally speaking, low-density drives behave unpredictably where high-density disks are concerned. That is, a low-density drive may properly read information from a high-density disk that has been formatted low but there is always a possibility of its refusing to read the disk at all; writing to such disks is unreliable at best.

Low-density 3.5-inch disks are designed to store 720K of data while their high-density counterparts hold 1.44MB. Again, high-density drives will automatically format disks high so that one must issue a special command line parameter in order to format a disk low. As in the 5.25 world, the high-density drives are capable of reading the 720K disks whereas the low-density drives cannot read the 1.44MB format. While formatting a 720K disk high does not result in the production of bad sectors with nearly the same frequency as does formatting a 360K disk high (partially due to the fact that one is not quadrupling but merely doubling the intended storage capacity), engaging in this type of "conservation" is still inadvisable. Often high-density drives will simply refuse to read low-density disks that have been formatted high.

Hard disks must, of course, be formatted as well before any information can be written to them, but unlike floppy disks, which are often reformatted two or three times before being discarded as unusable, a computer's hard or fixed disk is usually formatted only once. Preparing a hard disk for use is somewhat more complicated than formatting a floppy disk since the disk must first be initialized or "low-level formatted," partitioned, and then made bootable with a system format. Once this has been accomplished, the hard disk will be able to store vast amounts of information, from the operating system to applications to data. Today, most desktop computers are outfitted with a 30 to 40MB hard disk but recent reductions in price have seen many end users purchasing 80 to 200MB hard drives for their home computers. Operating systems such as OS/2 consume an inordinate amount of space on the hard disk and applications running under Windows and the like are extremely large as well. But hard disks not only offer their users more storage space than single or dual floppy drive systems; they are faster and far more efficient than floppies—a much improved technology.

CD-ROM

Another type of computer disk that gained popularity in the mid-1980s is the CD-ROM. Each of these high-capacity disks can hold up to 680MB of data. This figure (713,031,680 bytes) represents over 275,000 printed pages of text. Today many reference works and literary collections are available on CD-ROM. Although few institutions and even fewer individuals own the drives used to access the disks, as with most computer equipment, the growing popularity of this storage unit is contributing to vast reductions in price. It is likely that CD-ROMs will be in fairly common use throughout colleges and universities and perhaps even in the homes of end users by the mid-1980s.

As the name suggests, CD-ROMs are a type of read-only device. There is no way to write information to the disks and they are entirely unerasable. Perhaps their greatest shortcoming is in the sluggishness with which information is retrieved. Although CD-ROMs access information in the same way as standard hard disks, they do so at approximately one-fifth the speed.

Peripheral Devices

A peripheral is any external input/output device connected to the system unit via a communications port. Printers, speech synthesizers, scanners, and modems are all examples of computer peripherals. Internal synthesizers and modems are not typically referred to as peripherals, since they are mounted in expansion slots within the system unit. Modems are discussed below, while chapter 4 includes a detailed explanation of synthetic speech hard- and software. We will begin with a discussion of scanners.

Optical Character Recognition

Optical character recognition (OCR) is the process of scanning and recognizing images printed on a page. It is, therefore, a two-step process. Unlike text, graphics are scanned but not recognized. They are simply reproduced in what is called a bit-mapped format, i.e., a pixel-by-pixel, or dot-by-dot, duplication of the image's composite parts is stored electronically on computer disk. Our present concern will be entirely with text recognition, i.e., the process by which the bit-mapped image of the printed page is ultimately translated to meaningful text in an accessible format. Indeed, optical character readers (OCRs) procured for use by blind and visually impaired users should have the ability to remove graphics automatically, since more often than not, these graphic images will interfere with the print-impaired reader's comprehension of the scanned text.

Scanning simply involves the electronic reproduction of an image while recognition entails a complexity of pattern-matching procedures and contextual rules. A scanner is a peripheral hardware device that takes a picture of the printed page and then transmits this image via a communications port to the recognition software which resides on computer disk. Once the text has been recognized, it is generally stored in ASCII code. In this way, users may retrieve the file for later reference and review using any number of applications software and adaptive technologies. Moreover, the machine-readable text file may be used to produce braille or large-print hard copy.

Most librarians will be familiar with the Kurzweil Personal Reader (KPR) and its predecessor the Kurzweil Reading Machine (KRM). Neither of these units is truly a peripheral device since both are fully operational in standalone mode. While the KPR is easily interfaced with a PC via an RS232 serial port, the equipment is not dependent upon this interface unless the user wishes to retain a machine-readable copy of the text that is being scanned and recognized. The KPR is equipped with its own recognition software, text-to-speech program, and internal DECTalk synthesizer.

Today there are a number of popular optical character recognition systems specifically designed for use by print-impaired users. The Adhoc, the Arkenstone Reader, and OsCaR are all high-quality OCR systems that provide adaptive technology users with a friendly interface to both the scanning and recognition processes. Each of these peripheral units is versatile and, in many regards, offer their users far more flexibility than the KPR.[3]

When selecting an OCR device, one should verify that it is not only fully compatible with the access system or systems of choice but that it has a high resolution and can handle a broad range of fonts and text qualities as well. The scanner's resolution relates to the number of pixels or dots per inch (DPI) an image, once scanned, will be composed of. A high-resolution scanner will help augment accuracy during the recognition process since images composed of a greater number of DPI will be less likely to blur and break apart. A poor resolution scanner may cause the recognition software to make such errors as producing "cl" rather than "d," for example. Resolution factors of 300 to 400 DPI are generally quite good. All OCRs will have some limitations regarding the variety of fonts and point sizes they can handle accurately. Whether or not letter spacing is even or proportional may also influence an OCR's accuracy as will the text quality itself. One should, however, be wary of advertised accuracy since accuracy is always determined under the best of all possible conditions, i.e., taking that particular device's specific limitations into consideration. Thus, looking at accuracy alone may not be an adequate gage of an OCR's capabilities. A system that handles a broader range of fonts, point sizes, and text qualities but has a somewhat lower accuracy rate than a device that is limited in these areas may still be a better buy.

Aside from performance, one will also want to take the OCR's features into account before purchasing a system for use by the print-impaired. Can the device handle "landscape" (sideways) as well as "portrait" (vertical) text? Does it, as mentioned previously, remove graphics automatically? Can it still scan and recognize material that has been placed on the scanner upside down? Does it support an automatic document feeder? Do multiple column formats present difficulties for the recognition software? Each of these features will be of particular concern to the blind or visually impaired user who will have to rely upon the system's "intelligence" to a greater extent than the sighted user who can, for example, determine in advance whether or not a page is printed sideways, contains graphics or columns, and is properly oriented on the scanner.

Printers

A printer is an external output device that generally connects to the computer via a parallel port. Peripherals such as scanners, speech synthesizers, and mice are connected to one of the computer's serial ports where data are transmitted in asynchronous fashion over a single line. Parallel transmission of data is much faster since data are sent over multiple lines. With more than one line open, information need not be transmitted one character at a time.

There are basically three types of printers with which readers will probably be familiar: daisy wheel, dot matrix, and laser. Daisy wheel printers are similar to typewriters in that fully formed characters are produced when a rapidly rotating print element strikes the ribbon against the page. While these printers produce letter quality text, they cannot generate graphics, and making changes in size and appearance is extremely difficult since typeface and point size are dependent upon the element itself. Dot matrix printers have the advantage of enabling the production of graphics and text of varying sizes and styles since, as the name suggests, each character is composed of many tiny dots that can be altered on command.

If, however, the printer's resolution is poor, output may be fuzzy. Indeed, many OCRs will have difficulty with material produced by dot matrix printers.

Unlike daisy wheel and dot matrix printers, laser printers produce text page by page rather than character by character and do not employ an impact method. Rather, electrical impulses cause a laser beam inside the printer to scan a positively charged drum that is discharged wherever the beam hits. A fine black powder called toner is then applied to the drum, sticking only to the areas that have been discharged. As the drum rotates, the toner is deposited on the paper where a heating process seals the image. Laser printers have excellent resolution and can generate a wide array of typefaces, sizes, and graphics. Moreover, they will often use a page description language such as PostScript to enhance text quality even further. Using a sophisticated word-processing program such as WordPerfect and a laser printer, one can easily produce high-quality large print documents for use by individuals with low vision.

Whether or not a document is suitable for use by a patron having low vision will depend not only on the resolution or clarity of the print but, perhaps even more essentially, on the size of the characters themselves. Individual character height and the space between lines of text is measured in units called "points." One point is .0138 inch, so that there are 72 points to an inch. Standard print is 12 point. Large print generally is considered to start with characters printed in 14 points, but as this is only slightly larger than normal, most low-vision readers will benefit from 16- to 20-point text. One may also adjust "leading"—the amount of space between each line of text—to augment a document's overall readability. Although dot matrix printers can produce large print documents, problems inherent to poor resolution are amplified with each increase in point size. Thus, laser printers will yield the best results for uncommonly large lettering.

Despite the fact that the terms "font" and "typeface" are frequently used interchangeably, they are not synonymous. Point size is one aspect of a font; typeface is another. Each family of type is defined by an identifiable set of characteristics. Examples of families of type are Courier, Helvetica, and Times. Within each family are a variety of typefaces such as Times Roman, Times Bold, and Times Italic. While the underlying characteristics of each typeface within the family are the same, the design differs slightly from one to the other depending upon the particular weight and slant of the characters. A font is a set of characters printed in a particular typeface and of a specified size. Thus, 12-point Times Roman is a different font than 14-point Times Roman. A printer that supports several different fonts may not, therefore, be quite as versatile as one might think. A diversity of typefaces is what renders a printer's output unique. For our purposes, however, one would expect that the typefaces be "scalable," meaning that different point sizes could be selected at random.

Telecommunications and Networks

When two different computers are speaking to one another via telephone lines, they are engaging in telecommunications. In order for the computers to do this, both must be equipped with modems. A modem can be either an internal card that fits into one of the computer's expansion slots or an external device that plugs directly into a serial port. In either case, one of the computer's communications ports will be engaged. In order to use a modem, which is a hardware device, users must install telecommunications software such as ProComm, BitComm, or Telex. This software is what enables users to dial, connect, and actually communicate with a remote computer.

Modems transmit and receive information in analog format which is then redigitized for use by the local computer. The speed with which modems transmit data is measured in bits per second (BPS). Most modems in use on home computers today transmit at 1200 or 2400 BPS. This figure is also referred to as baud rate; however, baud and bps are not quite the same. Baud, derived from the name of an early French telegrapher, J. M. E. Baudot, is a generic term that denotes the number of discrete elements of data that can be transmitted in a given time frame. BPS is a far more limited term than baud, relating specifically to computer protocols.

Although online information services, electronic mail, and interactive bulletin boards are extremely popular with the general population of computer users, this form of information exchange can be of even greater use to print-impaired individuals. Machine-readable information "downloaded" (received) from a remote computer need not be modified for use by print-impaired users since it is preeminently accessible. Access to large databases, reference materials, and computerized card catalogs is equally empowering. There is, indisputably, a strong trend toward the use of electronic information since it can be stored or disposed of far more efficiently than that printed on paper, and it can be shared by a multiplicity of users simultaneously. Already in France, many people get their news and other daily information from computer terminals provided at low cost by the government. If the trend continues in this country as well, many blind, visually impaired, and learning-disabled users will surely benefit.

Networks also enable communication between two or more computers. A wide area network (WAN) is not restricted by geographic proximity. WANs may connect computers across cities, states, countries, and continents. A local area network (LAN), on the other hand, is bound by geographic proximity. Many businesses and colleges use LANs to allow computer workstations to share programs, data, and peripherals. Each of the workstations in a LAN is installed with a network card that enables communication with the file server and thus the network operating system. The file server is one of the computers in the network that has been designated to store community files and regulate operating system commands. The file server may be dedicated to its task or it may also act as a workstation. As LANs grow in size, the importance of maintaining a dedicated file server increases since user applications will slow the network down and augment the possibility of conflicts.

Conclusion

As one industry analyst put it, "The original PC and its offspring have been wonderful enabling technology. But technology by itself doesn't ignite change. People make change. People have to be smart enough to see potential and then be brave enough to do something about it."[4] There can be no doubt that the potential to resolve virtually all questions of access to print for blind, visually impaired, and learning-disabled readers currently exists within the computer world. The following chapters are dedicated to showing the reader just how that precious potential might be unleashed.

Notes

1. See chapter 4 for a more detailed discussion of expanded versus extended memory and the advantages of using the upper memory area with adaptive software packages.
2. See chapter 4 for a detailed discussion of the graphical user interface and the problems it engenders for speech-based adaptive technology.
3. See appendix B for a complete listing of adaptive technology products and vendors.
4. Cheryl Currid, "Corporate Reflections on the PC's 10th Birthday," *PC Week* 8 (Aug. 5, 1991): 64.

Chapter 3

Tactile Reading Methods and Materials

The earliest educators of the blind realized the importance of training their students to rely on the sense of touch to compensate for their inability to see. Using embossed educational materials, they demonstrated that blind people could be taught to read (and to write) as long as they had materials in a format accessible to them. This trend toward conversion of print into tactile media continued into the twentieth century, when technology engendered a number of auditory options to print, including "talking," or recorded, books, and, more recently, systems based on synthetic speech. These auditory methods never completely replaced touch reading (primarily of braille materials) for a number of reasons that will be set forth below. Today, many print-impaired individuals think of braille as just one of several options at their disposal for accessing the printed page.

In this chapter, we will investigate the history of touch reading and writing systems, clearing up, we hope, some misconceptions about braille, one of the earliest and certainly the most enduring of alternative reading methods available to the print-impaired reader. Many people immediately think of braille as the primary medium of information exchange available to blind and visually impaired people. However, while it remains the most popular touch reading system, braille has always had competition, and even today there are a few tactile reading alternatives in use by visually impaired individuals. In addition to braille materials and technology, we will consider the implications of one electronic touch reading system, the OptaCon (Optical to Tactile Converter), a device that emits a vibrating sensation on the tip of the reader's finger in the actual shape of numbers or letters of the alphabet.

Finally, we will explore in some detail the technology available for the local production of braille texts. Before undertaking production, however, most readers will want to find out if the desired title has already been produced in braille and if so, how a copy of the text might be acquired. We will then describe how libraries can do their own desktop publishing of material not otherwise available.

A General Look at Braille

The History of Braille

The idea of educating the blind has its intellectual and philosophical roots in the French Enlightenment.[1] Its real beginning, for all practical purposes, is often associated with the opening in 1784 of the Institut des Jeunes Aveugles, the first school devoted to the education of blind children. The movement to educate the blind soon spread from France to other countries of Europe, including England and Scotland, and gave rise to a number of "embossed alphabets." Based on the traditional (Roman) alphabet, these pre-braille tactile substitutes for print allowed the blind person to read by feeling the shapes, in relief, of actual letters, numbers, and marks of punctuation.[2]

Perhaps the most influential of the early educators of the blind in France was Valentin Haüy, founder of the Institut des Jeunes Aveugles in Paris. His system of raised type, based on the Roman alphabet and "the round hand that students were learning to write with the pen,"[3] represented one of the earliest attempts to create texts accessible to the blind. Pages of books were embossed, and students were taught to read with their fingers by feeling the actual shapes of the letters on the page. Needless to say, production of such embossed texts was enormously expensive, and there were very few titles in the library of the Institut des Jeunes Aveugles. However, with just a few books Haüy did manage to teach people with visual impairments to read, even if the shortage of materials available in this format must have been profoundly frustrating to these newly literate individuals.

Braille, a writing system that uses raised dots to represent numbers and letters of the alphabet, was developed by Louis Braille, a student at the Institut des Jeunes Aveugles, in 1829—just thirty-seven years after the introduction of Haüy's embossing process. The idea of using dots to represent numbers and letters was not actually invented by Braille, but was already in use in the "night-writing" code developed by Charles Barbier for the French army. Barbier used a rather arbitrary eight-dot cell configuration to facilitate communication on the dark battlefield; Louis Braille's more efficient system employed just six dots per cell, and is still used today as the tactile substitute for print by most of the world's languages.[4] Louis Braille's most significant contribution to the field of education of the visually impaired was the development of a code that was both abstract and systematic, i.e., very similar to print itself, which could be used not only for reading but as a method of writing as well. With the introduction of the braille code, true literacy—the ability to read *and* to write—became a possibility for blind and visually impaired people for the first time in history.

While many people still think of braille as the primary communication medium of blind and visually impaired people, this has not been the case since early in the twentieth century, when recorded, or "talking," books were introduced as an option. A number of technological and social phenomena continue to threaten the status of braille as the primary means of communication available to the blind reader. Audio technology (records and tapes) and, more recently, computer-based synthetic speech compete with braille as viable adaptive technologies for the blind and visually impaired. Optical character recognition technology, including scanners and intelligent reading machines, extend the options available for the translation of print into speech or other accessible output (including braille, as we will see in the section on in-house braille production, below).

A number of social forces have also had an effect on braille literacy. Primary among them is the trend to integrate children with visual disabilities into regular schools at all educational levels, from preschool through graduate and professional schools. In the nineteenth century and well into the twentieth, blind children typically attended special, often residential, schools for the blind where braille was usually taught. As a result of decades of "mainstreaming," children with visual disabilities are less likely to receive the extensive training in braille that they did when attending specialized schools, the use of braille being commonly replaced by human readers and audio technology.

Today, we are beginning to see the effects of mainstreaming extending in many directions beyond the classroom. Increasing numbers of people with disabilities attend universities and colleges and go on to pursue careers in fields that were, until recently, simply inaccessible to them. Blind, visually impaired, and learning-disabled college students need access—preferably independent access—to the same materials their sighted classmates and professors take for granted. This includes journals, monographs, and reference works that will not be available in braille in the college or university library; indeed, only a fraction of the student's required reading material can be found in braille anywhere in the world.

Two computer-based innovations are radically changing the availability of braille text. The first, the desktop braille printer, often called an "embosser," produces braille in paper copy. Braille printers, and their potential for use in libraries, will be discussed later in this chapter. Another innovation, the "soft," or "paperless" braille device, converts computer text, line by line, into synthetic speech or braille (on a reformable strip). Virtually anything that can be accessed via computer can be read on these devices, introducing an exciting new level of independence for blind and visually impaired individuals who want or need reading materials in braille.

Ironically, some of the new, PC-based technology, which once threatened the future of braille, may in fact be exerting a positive impact on the use and production of this communication medium. As Catherine Mack put it, "Technology can support, enhance, and promote braille literacy. Technology can increase the amount of braille reading material available, expand the variety of braille reading material available, create more immediate access to braille material, and facilitate braille note-taking."[5] For braille users, any increase in the amount and variety of braille publishing activity is very good news. Even more exciting is the ability of the blind to copy library books and other materials in braille almost as easily as the sighted population can photocopy them.

Plusses and Minuses of Braille

Each alternative to print has advantages and disadvantages in relation to each of the other formats. Braille texts, for example, are much more expensive to produce than recorded materials. Readers also frequently cite the bulkiness of braille as a serious disadvantage; the braille edition of the *Oxford Companion to French Literature*, a one-volume reference work in print, comprises twenty-three fairly thick volumes of braille. A typical braille volume occupies over six inches of shelf space, and has a rather cumbersome 12-by-12-inch binding. With the vast amount of information available and necessary in our day-to-day lives, it is very easy to see why recorded and machine-readable options are attractive to the blind or visually impaired reader.

There are, however, some undeniable advantages to braille, particularly as a medium of instruction. First of all, reading by touch is very similar to reading by sight. Reading a text in print or in braille requires deriving meaning from what is essentially an object; when we listen, on the other hand, we are experiencing language in a very different manner—a manner that does not require understanding of the conventions of print. Educators of the blind stress the important skills gained by "real reading" (as opposed to "listening")—skills such as mastery of spelling and grammar. Braille is an active reading process, as opposed to listening, and many educators fear the steadily increasing reliance on passive, auditory reading methods.[6] Details readers of print take for granted, such as paragraphing and other conventions of structure, might elude the blind reader who relies solely on auditory reading methods.

Historically, although some libraries developed special facilities for serving people with disabilities, few libraries have taken an active role in the collection or dissemination of braille texts. The bulkiness of braille, as well as the expense involved in the production of braille books and magazines, makes an extensive collection unmanageable for the typical library. In response to this situation, a network of special libraries for the blind (later extended to include the "physically handicapped"), the National Library Service, was organized by the Library of Congress. The National Library Service (NLS) is, today, the primary supplier of braille texts on a national level. The world's largest producer of braille as well as audio-format reading materials, the NLS will be discussed below in connection with the traditional braille production establishment.

Today, libraries with the capacity for computer-based desktop braille publishing can produce braille on demand. With the proliferation of machine-readable texts, full-text online, and CD-ROM sources, the number and variety of potentially accessible texts for braille readers is vast. Virtually any of these machine-readable texts can be printed in paper copy braille or read by touch with a refreshable braille computer display (discussed below).

Production of a paper copy braille text requires some work, but microcomputer technology has made the task manageable. However, while the cost of production has dropped, braille texts are still expensive to produce. Before undertaking production, therefore, the librarian serving the blind reader should attempt to locate a copy of the desired item already in braille. To convey to the reader what is involved in braille production, we will first try to explain how braille works and then investigate the braille publishing industry and its relationship to libraries.

The Mechanics of Braille

Grade 1 Braille

Each braille unit, commonly referred to as a "cell," is composed of six dots—two dots wide and three dots high, whether or not all six potential dots are present. That is, a single letter or contracted word form (discussed later in connection with grade 2 braille) might be represented by just one dot (as the letter a = $\vdots$); it is the *position* of this dot within the six dot configuration that identifies it as an a.

The alphabet and numerals 1 through 0 are illustrated in figure 1. Notice that the first ten letters of the alphabet, *a* through *j*, double as numerals 1 through 0. One of two special symbols precedes those cells that are to be read as numerals or symbols. This type of braille, commonly referred to as grade 1, is very similar to the original code as devised by Louis Braille. Louis Braille based his touch reading code on a "Principle of Logical Sequence." According to this principle, the first ten letters of the alphabet form the bases of all other letters and signs. Thus the eleventh letter, *k*, is an *a* with the addition of the lowest left-hand dot in the cell, and so on for the second ten letters, while the remaining letters of the alphabet are formed by adding a second dot on the bottom row. As the French alphabet contains no *w*, this letter was missing from Braille's original system. Introduced later to meet the needs of other

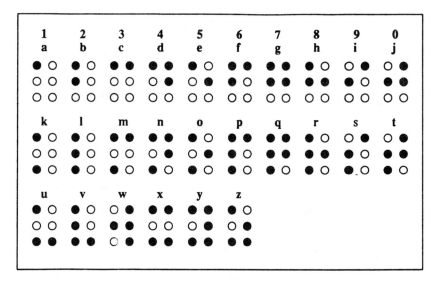

Figure 1. Grade 1 Braille alphabet and numbers

languages, it is formed from a *j* by the addition of the lowest right-hand dot of the cell.[7]

Grade 2 Braille

Grade 2 braille consists of grade 1, as well as close to two hundred contractions for frequently occurring word parts, such as suffixes and prefixes. In addition, each letter of the alphabet can represent a common word and, as mentioned above, the cells for the first ten letters of the alphabet also represent the numbers 1 through 0. For example, consider the three possible readings of the braille symbol for the letter *c*. If the symbol for the letter *c* stands alone in a line of text, the reader assumes that the symbol represents its *word* equivalent (in this case, the *c* represents the word "can"). However, if contextual clues are not sufficient to alert the reader to the meaning of a symbol, the cell is preceded by one of two special symbols that denote "number" or "letter." For example, in the sentence "I got a C in algebra this year," the braille cell for the letter *C* would be preceded by a symbol for letter. Similarly, the number 3 (which shares the configuration of the letter *c*) is preceded by the cell denoting number, so that the reader does not misinterpret the cell's meaning. Today, most braille readers expect grade 2 English braille; almost all publications produced by any of the major braille publishers (listed and described in appendix A) are produced in grade 2, contracted braille.

Figure 2 illustrates some of the contractions employed in grade 2 braille. It is easy to see how a much desired economy of space can be achieved

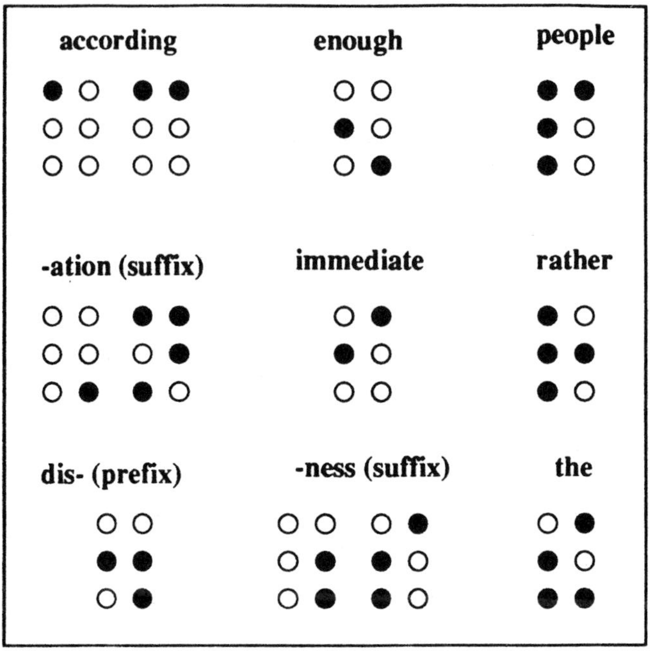

Figure 2. Examples of Grade 2 braille contractions (For a complete list of grade 2 braille contractions, see English Braille, American Edition, *1959 (American Printing House for the Blind, 1959)*

through the use of such contractions. In addition to rendering the text less bulky, the contractions of grade 2 braille permit much higher reading speeds, since considerably fewer cells are required to convey meaning.

One of the great boons to the popularity of braille came with the introduction of technology that permitted two-sided printing of texts. This process, which came to be known as "interpointing," results in a much less bulky (and, consequently, less expensive) braille text. Braille cells are spaced so that they fall between the cells on the reverse side of the page, making the text take just half the paper required by one-sided braille copy. Several of the computer-based braille printers profiled at the end of this chapter and listed in appendix B are capable of producing two-sided, interpointed braille texts.

Braille Writing

As noted above, braille's success as a written language is a result of the complete literacy it affords the user; that is, not only can braille be read, it can be written as well. Earlier embossed alphabets failed because they could not be written so easily. Letters of the Roman alphabet are, after all,

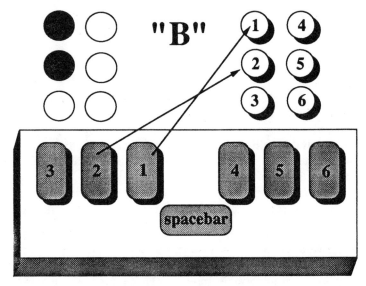

Figure 3. Braille keyboard layout. Letters and words are formed by depressing the key or keys that correspond to the cell's dots. By depressing keys 1 and 2 simultaneously, the braille cell representing the letter B is formed.

designed to be seen, and do not take into account the nature of touch reading and writing.

The use of slate and stylus for braille writing and note taking is a skill that is disappearing, but some people are still proficient in this type of writing. Basically, written braille is the mirror image of the braille code. The writer pokes dots into heavy paper, and the text is read from the other side. This involves writing backwards, from right to left, and reversing the configuration of dots for each character, number, or contraction. The symmetry of the braille code makes this a learnable system. The sighted reader might imagine how difficult it would be to have to write backwards; indeed, reversing the letters of the Roman alphabet would be difficult. Because of the simplicity, symmetry, and logical nature of the braille cell, however, the task of producing characters in reverse is made much less trying.

While few individuals still use slate and stylus to produce braille, many more are adept in the use of braille note-taking devices that employ braille "keyboards." Some of the "soft" or "refreshable" braille devices, described later in this chapter, use six keys—one for each of the braille cell's dots—as their input device. Figure 3 shows the correspondence between braille keyboard and braille cell. Requiring only six keys, many of these devices are extremely small, and become convenient notebooks and address books for their blind users. Some devices, like the Braille 'n Speak, offer synthetic speech output; others use a braille display strip with lines of braille "pins" that pop up in the form of braille text, and are replaced line by line with succeeding lines of text (hence the term "refreshable braille").

Braille Use

Literacy for print-impaired individuals has a short history, but that history is inextricably linked with braille. However, according to statistics gathered by the National Library Service, braille readership among registered library users has declined steadily over the past few decades. Some educators fear the consequences of the steady decline in braille literacy among the visually impaired population, and have proposed several reasons to explain it. One of the reasons often put forth by educators is the inadequate preparation of braille teachers. Karen Luxton of City University of New York explains:

> Braille hasn't been well taught, partly because there have been so few teachers trained in vision. Blind students typically encounter "generic special education" teachers who, if they've been exposed to braille at all, that exposure has been minimal. Reading by touch is fundamentally different from reading by listening. While you can actively listen, auditory methods are essentially "passive" reading methods. Braille is an *active* reading process. Braille users can master such print-based skills as spelling, punctuation, and important print-based structures, such as paragraphing."[8]

Another reason proposed for the decline in braille readership involves the scarcity of certain types of braille materials. Only a small fraction of the current publishing output is ever converted to braille. Estimates vary, but the number of titles mass-produced in braille in the United States each year is under 500, compared with an annual production of over 40,000 English language books. In fiscal year 1990, the National Library Service reports production of only 373 new mass-produced titles in braille, compared with 1,734 new cassette titles.[9] This relative scarcity of materials probably has an effect on the motivation of the blind to master braille to a significant degree. Remember also that people with visual impairments are pursuing higher levels of education than ever before, entering fields in which very little of the professional literature has ever been produced in braille.

It may be true that changes in society and the demographics of blindness, as well as the availability of options for the print-impaired reader, have chipped away steadily at braille use. However, the importance of braille continues to be argued by national organizations concerned with the welfare of the blind, and some observers foresee an increase in the amount and variety of braille texts. Any increase in access to braille materials will certainly help to secure the viability of braille as an important reading medium for the blind.

Braille Publishing and the Role of Libraries

Braille books and periodicals are produced by several publishers, many of which were at one time associated with schools for the blind. One such publisher, the American Printing House for the Blind (APH), today the world's largest producer of educational texts in braille, was originally the print shop for the Kentucky School for the Blind.[10] The efforts of these organizations are coordinated by the National Library Service of the Library of Congress, which supplies materials through a network of regional libraries.

Braille has always held a unique place in the structure of libraries. Typically, libraries collect materials from outside sources, the commercial publishing industry being the largest. But because of the enormous expense associated with the production of braille texts, "commercial production has never been feasible. The demand—further reduced in the early days by the multiplicity of touch-reading codes in use—has always been too small for profitable mass production. The cost and sheer bulk of braille materials precluded personal collections, hence the great need for lending libraries for adults once the education of blind children was well under way."[11]

The National Library Service

While there were some individual libraries serving patrons with disabilities as early as the 1890s, the beginning of a coordinated national effort to provide library service to disabled people began in 1931 with the creation of the National Library Service for the Blind (NLS) of the Library of Congress; passage of the Pratt-Smoot Act in that year guaranteed annual federal funds for the production and dissemination of embossed books geared toward the adult blind population. By 1952, the program was extended to include service to children as well. In 1966, eligibility for NLS service was further extended to include individuals diagnosed with physically based learning disabilities. Anyone who cannot hold, handle, or read conventional printed materials because of a physical disability is eligible for library service through a national network of libraries cooperating with the renamed National Library Service for the Blind and Physically Handicapped. Materials available through the NLS include braille, "talking books" (in both disk and cassette tape formats), and large print. Talking books and large print materials are discussed in chapters 4 and 5 respectively.

NLS serves as the national clearinghouse for texts in braille and other formats accessible to readers with print impairments. Through a network of fifty-six regional and ninety-two subregional libraries, materials are mailed, postage free, to qualified individuals or institutions (such as libraries, nursing homes, and hospitals). Funded annually by Congress, the FY 1990 appropriation totaled $37,112,000 for materials and services. In addition to federal funds, most regional and subregional libraries receive support from state and, in some cases, local government budgets.

In addition to producing recorded and braille reading materials, the NLS makes available, on loan, the special playback equipment required to use audio format texts. Network regional and subregional libraries supply space, library personnel, and all other aspects of service to their local clientele. The NLS also coordinates the training and placement of volunteers, who represent an important aspect of service to the target population.

NLS Collections

Books and magazines are chosen for inclusion in the collection of the National Library Service on the basis of their appeal or importance to the widest possible audience. "Bestsellers, biographies, fiction and how-to books are in great demand. Titles expected to be extremely popular are produced on flexible disk in several thousand copies and circulated to borrowers within several months of their publication in print form."[12] Highly specialized, professional, or educational materials (textbooks) are expressly not produced or collected by the National Library Service. Rather, the National Library Service should be thought of as the equivalent of the local public library, whose collections are geared toward the general reader.

Foreign-language reading materials, primarily Spanish-language texts, make up a growing segment of the collection. In addition to Spanish, languages represented in the mass-produced foreign-language collection include French, Italian, German, Portuguese, Polish, Laotian, and Vietnamese.[13] As of January 1991, the NLS collections contained thirteen million items comprising 59,000 titles. In 1990, braille and recorded and cassette books and magazines were circulated by NLS to a total readership of 659,350. The average reader borrows thirty recorded books and magazines a year, with braille readers averaging an additional thirty titles per year.[14]

In addition to books and magazines in braille and recorded formats, NLS provides the playback equipment, free of charge, to users registered for service. Talking Book machines, which were developed for the National Library Service, play recorded disk materials at speeds of 8 or 16 rpm. Special cassette tape playback machines designed specifically for NLS cassettes are also available free of charge to individuals and institutions registered with the National Library Service. NLS audio playback equipment will be discussed in much greater detail in chapter 4.

NLS: Eligibility of Individuals

In order to qualify for service, individuals or organizations must submit an application, available from any library in the NLS network. (For a complete list of network libraries, contact the National Library Service or the regional/subregional library in your area.)

Services are available under the following conditions of eligibility:

A. The following persons are eligible for loan service:
   1. Blind persons whose visual acuity, as determined, is 20/200 or less in the better eye with correcting lenses, or whose widest diameter of visual field subtends an angular distance no greater than 20 degrees.
   2. Other physically handicapped persons as follows:
      a. Persons whose visual disability, with correction and regardless of optical measurement, is certified by competent authority as preventing the reading of standard printed material.
      b. Persons certified by competent authority as unable to read or unable to use standard printed material as a result of physical limitations.
      c. Persons certified by competent authority as having a reading disability resulting from organic dysfunction and of sufficient severity to prevent their reading printed material in a normal manner.
B. In cases of blindness, visual disability, or physical limitations, "competent authority" is defined to include doctors of medicine, doctors of osteopathy, ophthalmologists; optometrists; registered nurses; therapists; professional staff of hospitals, institutions, and public or welfare agencies (e.g., social workers, case workers, counselors, rehabilitation teachers, and superintendents). In the absence of any of these, certification may be made by professional librarians or by any person whose competence under specific circumstances is acceptable to the Library of Congress.
C. In the case of reading disability from organic dysfunction, competent authority is defined as doctors of medicine and doctors of osteopathy who may consult with colleagues in associated disciplines.
D. Qualified readers must be residents of the United States, including the several states, territories, insular possessions, and the District of Columbia, or American citizens domiciled abroad.

(Source: Library of Congress, National Library Service for the Blind, *Application for Free Library Service: Individuals*)

NLS: Eligibility of Institutions

Virtually any library can act as an information and referral service for blind and visually impaired individuals. Interested librarians should contact their local or regional NLS library for details. For libraries serving patrons who are registered for service with NLS, equipment such as NLS flexible disk and cassette playback equipment may be borrowed free of charge. Such libraries will also qualify for free subscriptions to the major NLS publications, such as *Braille Books* and *Talking Book Topics*. The National Library service has produced a number of other reference circulars and bibliographies on disabilities; see appendix C for a list of publications produced by the NLS and other agencies.

For libraries interested in providing information and referral services to their print-impaired clientele, an important first step will be the establishment of a collection of materials on diverse disabilities. Each of the associations and publishers identified in appendix A can provide literature in accessible media on a variety of disabilities. The NLS reference circular *Building a Library Collection on Blindness and Physical Handicaps: Basic Materials and Resources*, last updated in 1986, provides a good list of core books and periodicals on disabilities.

Volunteer Organizations

While the activities of the National Library Service are funded annually by Congress, the services of individuals as well as groups of volunteers are an important component of the overall program of library service to print-impaired individuals. According to the NLS, "volunteers produce a wide variety of braille and recorded materials for visually and physically disabled readers. They may transcribe such varied items as a textbook for a college student, a series of Supreme Court decisions for a lawyer, or a bestselling novel for a general reader."[15]

Since 1943, the National Library Service has acted as the national clearinghouse for information on groups and individuals who provide volunteer library services to people with disabilities. Its *Volunteers Who Produce Books*, published every two to three years as needed, lists organizations and individuals who produce reading materials in braille, recorded formats, and large print. Arranged by state, and further subdivided by city or town, *Volunteers Who Produce Books* includes a subject index where one might identify individuals or groups equipped to produce specialized braille texts such as science, math, or foreign-language materials. Special supplements include a list of Special Education Resources as well as a Register of Certified Proofreaders, also arranged by state.

The impact of volunteers on the overall quality of service to people with disabilities is inestimable; unfortunately, there are no reliable statistics available on the actual number of people involved in volunteer service. In a 1980 study on the role of volunteers within the overall NLS program of service, however, the "net volunteer contribution (gross worth minus administration costs) was set at a minimum of $3 million."[16] In 1992, according to John Wilkinson, Literary Braille Advisor at the National Library Service, there are at least 23,000 volunteers providing services to readers in need of special format texts.[17] The Braille Development Section of the NLS adds twenty braille transcribers to the NLS roster of volunteers each month. In addition to providing braille texts for the general NLS clientele, the nation's 23,000 volunteers transcribe an estimated 90 percent of all the textbooks used by blind students in the United States.[18]

Volunteers interested in producing hand-copied braille texts must pass a correspondence course and examination administered by the National Library Service. The course in literary braille, which is prerequisite to the more specialized courses offered by NLS, begins with an overview of the alphabet and culminates in specialized training in text formatting. Prospective braille transcribers must achieve a minimum grade of 80 on a final braille manuscript in order to be certified by the Library of Congress.[19] The Braille Development Section, which administers the correspondence courses leading to certification, offers advanced training in music, mathematics, and proofreading braille to students who have successfully completed the literary braille course. Volunteers interested in producing math or science texts must fulfill the requirements for certification in the Nemeth Code, a specialized six-dot tactile code designed for technical disciplines. Similarly, individuals interested in producing music materials receive training in a specialized notation for their discipline.[20]

Who benefits from the efforts of volunteer braille transcribers? Remember that, even with other options available, braille is still the most appropriate print substitute in many contexts. The braille literate reader who needs an advanced calculus textbook, for example, will most likely opt for a braille edition, rather than a tape recording. Similarly, students of foreign languages might require special grade one, letter-for-letter transcriptions of textbooks. Before they can effectively read or write contracted word forms, foreign-language learners must attain proficiency in the written language, which can only come from a complete knowledge of the word structure and orthography of the language in question.

Even libraries working with extremely limited financial resources can assist their blind and visually impaired patrons in locating volunteer transcribers for such projects. *Volunteers Who Produce Books*, the register of certified transcribers, should be considered an essential resource for the library providing information and referral services to their visually impaired clientele.

Locating Braille Texts

To assist the patron in the selection of materials, the National Library Service produces several reference sources to braille publications. Most NLS publications, such as *Braille Book Review* (bimonthly; see appendix C), which provides announcements and annotations of new titles in braille, are available free of charge to individuals and institutions registered for service. *Braille Books* is the *annual* list of braille titles produced by or available on loan from the National Library Service. Included in these listings are books brailled by NLS as well as those acquired by the National Library Service from other publishers.

Like most libraries, large and small, the NLS and some of its affiliated network libraries maintained card catalogs until relatively recently. Supplemented by book catalogs that provided subject access for very broad categories, these catalogs were cumbersome to use, and many catalogs had to be consulted in order to identify the existence of a desired item within the NLS system. The NLS claims that "in 1954 this situation was remedied to an extent when NLS began distributing to network libraries card catalog sets for each new mass-produced title. While a step forward, this did nothing to improve access to limited-production books such as those in handcopied braille, or to improve access to older material."[21]

In the 1970s, the National Library Service began automating its bibliographic records. Using a modified MARC format with certain fields adapted to describe items in the NLS holdings of special format materials, NLS staff began automated cataloging of braille and recorded book titles with the goal of producing a true union catalog of the system's holdings. Pieces of descriptive information specific to the accessible media under consideration were assigned their own MARC fields—for example, "sex of narrator" was indicated by a code in field 008: FF81. Other adapted MARC tags included cataloging source code (FF90), additional content information (FF82), and narrator added entry (code 790).

The NLS states that "by 1977, the first microfiche edition of the Union Catalog was produced and distributed to the network of cooperating libraries. The first fiche catalog contained records for 10,000 books."[22] Regional and subregional libraries in the NLS network continue to receive the microfiche version of *Reading Materials for the Blind and Physically Handicapped*, the cumulative union catalog of the National Library Service. Updated quarterly, this com-fiche catalog includes records of braille, recorded, and large print items available on loan from the NLS. The cumulative microfiche catalog offers seven access points to the holdings of the National Library Service. Indexes provide access to materials by author, title, subject, Dewey decimal classification number, foreign-language code, and narrator. "An appendix to the fiche contains a listing by title of NLS books still in production. This list, derived from the Production Control Section database, is especially useful for institutions that are planning to produce books and wish to avoid duplicating NLS efforts."[23] As increasing numbers of small publishers, libraries, and even individuals are beginning to produce titles in braille, the Union catalog, including the "books still in production" (a kind of *Forthcoming Accessible Books*), should be consulted before production begins so that costly duplication of effort can be avoided.

One of the last hurdles to independent access to libraries and their collections by disabled patrons is the ability to independently search the online catalog and other computerized information sources. A recent policy statement by the American Foundation for the Blind deplores the level of dependence required by the disabled user to gain access to library materials: "Despite the proliferation of database systems, the reading needs of blind and visually handicapped people rely . . . on an informal system of literature search that is usually dependent on the help of sighted persons."[24] With new technology, libraries are in a position to relieve this level of dependence upon the librarian. As this monograph goes to print, plans are well underway for the conversion of the NLS catalog from com-fiche to CD-ROM. With quarterly updates planned, this reference tool is being designed to allow for maximum independent access by print-impaired library users. "Equipped with a user-friendly interface, the CD-ROM version of the catalog will provide the option of independent searching by the library patron of the complete holdings of the NLS by subject, title, keyword and format."[25] In the next section, we will see that individuals and organizations are now producing braille texts; these too can be listed in the Union Catalog, if available for loan to patrons eligible for NLS service.

> The more materials listed, the more useful the Union Catalog will be to blind and physically handicapped users. NLS invites all who produce and/or maintain collections of braille and recorded books to send in their listings. Books must be held in a specific location and be available for loan or purchase when required by borrowers. NLS assumes the cost of cataloging. Information must be in a form that can be used for the Union Catalog. Contact the NLS Bibliographic Control Section for guidelines.[26]

The online version of the NLS catalog, BLND, is already available as a private database to qualified BRS users. Just about any library serving the blind or visually impaired community is eligible to search BLND. Of course, BLND is not free, but carries a charge like other BRS databases. In order to add BLND to your options as a BRS user, the National Library Service must approve the request. BRS subscribers should contact the National Library Service or their BRS representative for information about access to BLND.

The Reference Section of the National Library Service has developed a *Searchers' Manual* (print, recorded, and braille formats) for searchers of BLND. The manual, available from NLS free of charge to BLND searchers, is very clearly written and well organized, and is highly recommended for potential searchers of this fairly complex database. We're all familiar with the advantages of online searching; among the most beneficial aspects for the braille user are searches limited by *format*. Subject bibliographies of braille titles can be produced fairly inexpensively, and for the library equipped with a braille printer, these bibliographies can be edited and produced in braille.

The American Printing House for the Blind, founded in 1858 and supported by federal funds to provide educational materials for visually impaired students at all levels, also makes its online catalog available. APH-CARL (American Printing House-Central Automated Resource Listing) provides librarians and other professionals serving the information needs of blind and visually impaired individuals with online access to the holdings of APH. Accessible via computer using a modem and telecommunications software, APH-CARL is compatible with many adaptive computer devices, affording the visually impaired user independent access to the holdings of APH. Like NLS, the American Printing House for the Blind produces publications in audio formats as well as in braille. Remember, however, that the APH inventory is limited to educational materials, primarily elementary and secondary level textbooks.

NLS and APH are the major producers of braille in the United States. For a directory of other publishers of braille texts, see appendix A.

Other Touch Reading Codes

Prior to the international acceptance of the braille code in the twentieth century, numerous other tactile reading systems were in use throughout Europe and the United States. Some of these systems were modifications of the Roman alphabet, while others employed embossed dots or lines in a variety of configurations. In order to effectively use all of the embossed reading material published in the United States in the early part of the twentieth century, the literate blind had to learn numerous raised dot and other embossing systems, and many were believed to have stopped reading entirely because of the dearth of materials available in any one format. Radically different regional tactile systems, such as New York Point and Boston Line, had to be mastered for the blind reader to access publications produced in geographically diverse areas. In 1837, the first title produced entirely in braille, *L'Histoire de France*, was produced by the Institut des Jeunes Aveugles. It wasn't until almost a century later that a single version of braille was accepted as a standard by American and British authorities concerned with education of the blind.[27]

Other than braille, the only major tactile reading system still in use is Moon Type. Moon Type found proponents among those readers with limited sensitivity in their fingertips. Many individuals who lose their vision in old age, or as a result of a stroke or diabetes, lack the requisite sensitivity in their fingertips to make braille use feasible, or enjoyable, as a reading method. The history of Moon Type is almost as long as that of braille. Invented in 1847 and named for its inventor, Dr. William Moon of Brighton, England, Moon Type is a radically simplified tactile variant of the Roman alphabet. As such, it requires less training, and is particularly popular with older, adventitiously blind adults who are not about to invest the time and energy required to learn braille. Moon Type always had its largest audience in England, where titles in this format are still produced. While the NLS can supply some titles in Moon Type, publications in this format comprise just a tiny fraction of NLS offerings compared with braille, audio cassette, and flexible disk books and magazines.

Another electronic device worth mentioning here in connection with tactile reading is the Optacon Reading System. Invented in the late 1960s by John G. Linvill of Stanford University, the Optacon is a marvel of advanced electronic engineering. The Optacon uses piezoelectric crystals to convert printed text into a form that can be felt by the reader. The inspiration for Linvill's use of piezoelectric crystals to interpret the printed page came from an experience he had while on sabbatical in Germany. There he observed a "high-speed printer that printed letters with a small array of pins which were made to vibrate axially, forming letters by electromechanically driving only certain pins against a ribbon and the page."[28] The Optacon Reading System operates in much the same way, conveying the image of a printed letter or symbol into a tactile form that can be felt with one finger. Like earlier embossed alphabets, the Optacon is faithful to the alphabet. This is not always an advantage when it comes to training, particularly with readers who are not thoroughly familiar with the alphabet. Many users who rely heavily or exclusively on braille, for example, may not know the shapes of the letters of the alphabet, or may not know them well enough to develop an acceptable reading speed without considerable practice.

For many blind readers, however, the Optacon provides an unprecedented degree of independence once its operation is mastered. The reader places the index finger in a small scanner that, when moved across a line of text, emits electronic pulses to the fingertip in the shape of actual letters on the page. The ability to decode print provides the reader with the ability to read, independently, printed materials of all kinds. Effective use of the Optacon requires a considerable amount of training, and is not suitable for all visually impaired people. Again, while few libraries offer access to the Optacon, it is important for us to be aware of the range of options available to our readers so that we can provide materials in the appropriate format(s). How many librarians would expect a totally blind patron to seek regular print materials? Those who use the Optacon, as well as those who have access to other character recognition technologies and reading machines, will be able to make use of most of the library's regular print resources.

Production of Braille

The introduction of the personal computer in the 1980s has dramatically affected the types of services libraries can offer their print-impaired readers. For the braille reader, the advances associated with PC-based technologies are analogous to the invention of movable type for the print reader. Virtually anything that can be accessed by computer can be printed in braille, or read with a paperless braille device. Before describing the process and technologies available for production of braille in hard copy, we will examine the implications of the paperless braille device. While few libraries provide access to such equipment, the development of paperless braille is expected to have a very powerful impact on braille use and literacy.

Paperless Braille

Paperless braille devices comprise two related but different types of technology: braille output displays and "notetakers." Paperless braille displays, often called "soft" or "refreshable braille displays," convert a fixed portion of the computer screen into braille, usually in the form of a portion of a single line of text. Pins move up and down, forming braille cells which correspond to a fixed portion of the screen, and are replaced with each succeeding line of text.

Braille notetakers feature a braille display, braille keyboard, and varying amounts of internal memory. They essentially operate like self-contained word processors. The biggest advantage to the braille notetaker equipped with synthetic speech output is cost and maintenance. Smaller and significantly less expensive than a laptop computer, paperless braille notetakers make the perfect address book, notebook, etc.

Very few libraries provide access to paperless braille devices, but it is important for librarians to be aware of the full range of adaptive facilities their clients may be using. This is true not only with braille but with other technologies as well. In a recent survey by the Association of Research Libraries, some academic and research libraries do include a paperless braille device in their inventory of adaptive computer equipment, but these libraries are by far the exception.[29] One such device, the Navigator, converts the characters on the computer screen to braille. On a tactile display strip, pins move up and down, creating a temporary line of braille text, which changes with each line of text on the computer screen. One of the major drawbacks associated with braille is the bulkiness of texts in this medium; computer-based paperless braille devices have overcome this barrier and will undoubtedly continue to affect the use and popularity of braille in the future. For an annotated list of some popular soft braille devices, including the Navigator, see appendix B.

Desktop Braille Publishing Technology
Translation Programs

While few libraries will include soft braille devices among their list of adaptive devices, many more provide access to the technology required for the production of hard copy braille texts. We conclude our discussion of braille production with a survey of technologies available for the rapid in-house production of paper copy braille.

Even with the dramatic reduction in price associated with much of the technology described below, hard copy braille production is still expensive. Before undertaking production of an item in braille, therefore, readers and librarians will attempt to locate a copy already in braille. With the aid of translation programs and braille embossers, however, readers are not limited to the choices offered by the National Library Service or other producers of braille. The braille-related technology that has emerged with the development of the personal computer offers the braille reader the potential of converting just about any printed material into paper copy braille.

Braille Production

PC-based production of a braille text begins with a machine-readable file in ASCII format. ASCII code is described in chapter 2, in connection with the development of the personal computer and related technologies. Very briefly, each letter, number, mark of punctuation, etc., is assigned a unique numerical equivalent, an ASCII symbol. These symbols, or ASCII codes, form the raw material of text-based computer systems. This numerical code is typically converted to a print display on the computer screen by a text editor, such as WordPerfect or other word-processing software. It has been shown that the visible screen can be bypassed completely, and that the user may opt for speech to convey the contents of a computer screen. For the braille user, the same file can be sent directly to a paper copy braille printer, described below. Before printing, however, the file usually undergoes a translation process, from grade 1, or computer braille, to the contracted form of braille known as grade 2. Braille translation programs are described below, following an analysis of other potential sources of computer-based braille print.

Sources of Electronic Texts

When an item is not available in braille (and this is usually the case), identifying the item on a CD-ROM or online source can be the next best thing. When we save the results of a literature search on Dialog, BRS, or other bibliographic network, we are saving the file as an ASCII text file. The proliferation of full-text electronic sources in recent years has dramatically increased the potential amount of material available to the braille user. Dialog, BRS, and other major vendors of online databases offer access to an ever-increasing number of full-text sources. For braille users, the prospect of retrieving not only citations but also the text of articles in machine-readable form opens many new possibilities for independence. No longer hampered by the limited output of our major national producers of braille texts, readers who rely on braille, such as those who are both deaf and blind, can perhaps for the first time in history consider the study of subjects for which materials were, in the past, scant at best. Full-text searches of newspaper, journal, or encyclopedia articles, retrieved online and saved on a floppy disk, are easily converted to braille as described below (see figure 4).

A series of electronic text projects begun in the late 1980s also holds great potential for extending the number and types of sources available to the print-impaired reader who needs braille output. Project Gutenberg is one such program. The goal of Project Gutenberg, available on the Internet, is to make available ten thousand books in ASCII format by the year 2000. As of April 1992, Project Gutenberg offered free access to approximately fifty electronic texts, or "e-texts," already in the form required for conversion to braille.

Another type of publication that might be considered for production in braille are those produced by the library itself. Most libraries publish information bulletins and guides to their services and programs; many libraries also offer subject-specific reference guides, or pathfinders, to the materials in their collections. If produced on a computer, these too are good candidates for production in braille. What better way to promote and extend the accessibility of the library, and the library's commitment to serving their disabled clientele, than through the library's own publications?

Texts that cannot be located in machine-readable form must be scanned, using the OCR technology described in chapter 2. Interestingly, most texts are produced in machine-readable form, but are then rendered inaccessible by the traditional publishing industry. Presumably, most contemporary authors and scholars use computers, and submit their texts to a publisher on computer disk. At New York University, staff at the Center for Students with Disabilities have obtained floppy disk copies of texts directly from the authors for production of books in braille. In one case, a student who is both deaf and blind was provided access to a five-hundred-page text because of the author's willingness to supply a copy of the title on floppy disk.

Conversion of Print to Machine-Readable Text

While the number of full-text machine-readable information sources seems to be growing exponentially, not all texts exist, or are accessible, in computer form. Books, newspapers, and journal articles that are available exclusively in print form must be scanned and saved as an ASCII text file in order to be converted to braille.

We emphasize the importance of locating "ready-to-go" machine-readable sources because of some problems inherent in the nature of scanning. First, scanning is usually the most time-consuming aspect of braille production; using a Kurzweil Personal Reader for scanning, for example, each page of a book may take up to ninety seconds to scan; a fifty-page chapter of a book, at this rate, requires one and one-quarter hours of staff time at the scanner.

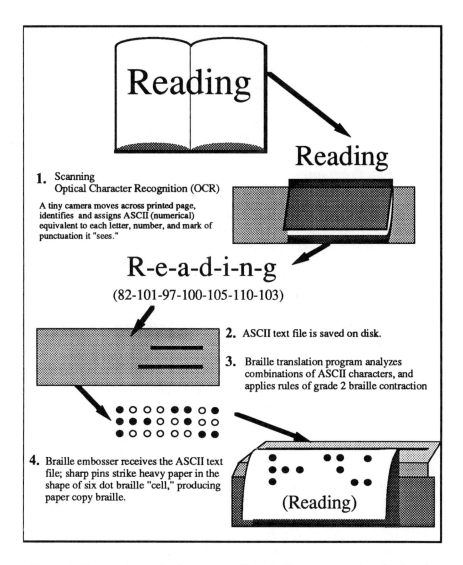

1. **Scanning**
   Optical Character Recognition (OCR)

   A tiny camera moves across printed page, identifies and assigns ASCII (numerical) equivalent to each letter, number, and mark of punctuation it "sees."

   R-e-a-d-i-n-g
   (82-101-97-100-105-110-103)

2. ASCII text file is saved on disk.

3. Braille translation program analyzes combinations of ASCII characters, and applies rules of grade 2 braille contraction

4. Braille embosser receives the ASCII text file; sharp pins strike heavy paper in the shape of six dot braille "cell," producing paper copy braille.

   (Reading)

Figure 4. The word "reading" is used to illustrate the processes involved in the production of grade 2 braille text, from scanning to embossing.

Second, scanned print materials are rarely 100 percent accurate. Depending on the quality of the scanning device as well as the clarity of the print being scanned, error rates may be as high as 15 percent per page. Consequently, a considerable amount of time can be required to proofread and edit a text of any length.

Some scanners, such as the OsCaR profiled in chapter 2, provide convenient "markers," which identify potentially misread text. That is, if the scanner is not sure, within certain parameters, of the identify of a character, it will insert a query symbol, such as "$" in OsCaR's case. This can greatly reduce the amount of time required for proofreading a scanned item. If edited with word-processing programs such as Word-Perfect, the proofreader can use the search command and go instantly from one problem word to the next.

Once the file has been saved on disk, it is ready to undergo the translation from grade 1, letter for letter, to grade 2, contracted braille.

Translation Programs

The development of sophisticated software for the conversion of texts to grade 2 braille has made possible the in-house production of paper copy braille. These software programs analyze the relationships between the letters and words in a computer file and apply abbreviated forms where appropriate. Remember that grade 2 braille uses close to two hundred contractions, and that these contractions are only applicable in strictly defined linguistic environments. The abbreviated symbol for the suffix ment (as in "apartment") for example, cannot be substituted for the *m-e-n-t* in the word "menthol." Rather, the symbol for the letter *m*, contractions for *en* and *th* followed by the symbols for the letters *o* and *l* comprise the grade 2 form of the word "menthol" (see figure 5). Remember also that in addition to these morpheme level rules, the symbols for the first ten letters of the alphabet double as numbers (e.g., ⠃ , the symbol for the letter *b*, can also represent the number 2); the number 2 would be preceded by a cell identifying it as a numeral.

The contracted, grade 2 text is then formatted for braille, and this file is sent to the braille embosser for printing. In addition to documents created with popular word-processing programs, such as WordPerfect or WordStar, files saved to disk from online sources or downloaded from a CD-ROM source can just as easily undergo the translation process.

There are several programs available that can rapidly apply the rules of contraction required for production of grade 2 braille. Foreign-language translation tables are also available for some programs. See appendix B for a directory and description of some popular braille conversion software programs.

In choosing a braille translation program, there are several points to consider:

- With which computers can the program interact? Is it compatible with any or all systems already in place?
- Is the translator compatible with the synthetic speech program (if any)?
- Can the translation program work with documents created with major word-processing software, such as WordPerfect?
- How easily can the user interface with the program?

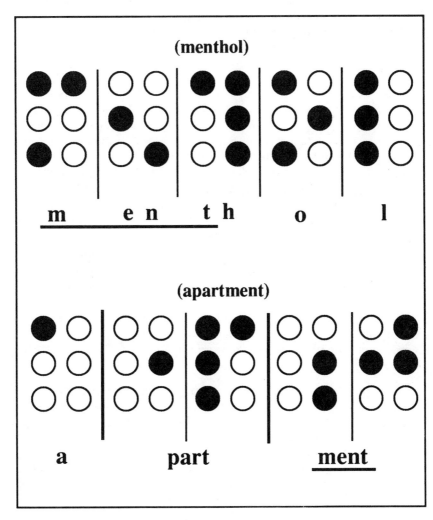

Figure 5. Linguistics of grade 2 braille contraction. Note the difference between "ment" in the words "menthol" and "apartment."

- How user friendly is the documentation? Is it available in accessible formats, such as cassette, tape, braille, or disk?
- Are options available for conversion of foreign-language materials?
- Can the program handle special materials, such as mathematics (Nemeth Code) and music?

When considering the purchase of a particular translation program, be aware of all specifications of the software and hardware with which the translator is expected to work. Of course, if the library has personnel who are knowledgeable in microcomputer technology, they should assist in selection of the braille translation program as they should with the purchase of any assistive peripheral hardware or software.

Braille Printers

Computer-based braille printers, sometimes referred to as "embossers," provide paper copy braille output of computer files. Mechanically, they all work in much the same way. A row of movable pins pops up in the shape of braille cells, striking heavy paper from behind and creating lines of braille text. However, while the mechanics are much the same, not all braille printers offer the same features. The Braille BookMaker, for example, can produce *interpointed* braille copy. Interpointing, as mentioned earlier, describes the process of creating double-sided braille copy. The braille cells on either side of the paper are placed so that they do not interfere with the other side, but are "interpointed," or placed between the points on the other side. The largest ongoing expense incurred in braille production is the cost of paper, and with the bulkiness of braille, texts can become quite costly. Interpointing will reduce the amount of braille paper used by 50 percent, resulting in a much less bulky text.

Other important features, such as printing speed, noise level, and technical support and documentation should be considered before purchasing the braille printer. The following questions might form the basis for selection of a paper copy braille printer:

1. What are the printer's special features? Can the printer produce two-sided, or interpointed, braille copy? Can the printer produce graphics or just text? Can a keyboard be attached directly to the printer, making it operate as a kind of typewriter?
2. How fast is the printer?
3. Is the printer user-friendly? Consider the needs of your disabled clientele here. Are the controls labeled with braille or other tactile symbols? Is there a logic to the arrangement of controls? How easy is it to load paper?
4. How noisy is the printer? All braille printers are noisy, given the nature of what they're doing. Optional acoustic enclosures are available for

some braille printers to alleviate the effect of the printer's noise level. If the printer is intended to be used in a room where other activities might be going on (such as listening to a reading machine or tape recorder), the sound enclosure will probably be mandatory. Before committing to a purchase, be sure to hear the printer with its enclosure. Even enclosed, the noise level of some printers will disallow other uses for the room in which it is placed. In a multiuse center, certain low-use times might be designated for braille printing.

5. Does the printer have a buffer, and how large is it? Braille printers with a large buffer can receive a large document, and free the host computer for other work. This can be important in multiuse centers, where the braille printer's host computer might have other output options—such as synthetic speech used for a variety of other purposes.

Some of the more popular braille printers are listed and described in appendix B.

Conclusion

Braille can be very useful as a medium of language instruction and transcription. Disadvantages such as the bulkiness of the text and the restricted titles available are being reduced by technological advances in the computer industry. The devices and programs we have discussed in this chapter will enable most libraries to expand enormously the services they can offer to their print-impaired patrons. The ready availability of almost any printed material transcribed into braille will no doubt contribute to an expansion in the braille literacy of the visually impaired.

Notes

1. With the publication of his *Lettre sur les Aveugles* in 1749, Diderot is credited with initiating an interest in the blind and with laying the foundations for the empirical study of blindness.
2. Elizabeth M. Harris, "Inventing Printing for the Blind," *Printing History* 8 (1986): 17.
3. Blind people were taught to write centuries before any large-scale attempt was made to teach complete literacy. The earliest account of writing education among the blind "is probably Harsdorffer's in his *Deliciae Mathematicae et Physicae*, published in Nurnberg in 1651, which describes a method of writing on wax tablets." (Charles G. Ritter, "Devices to Aid the Blind," in *Blindness: Modern Approaches to the Unseen Environment*, edited by Paul E. Zahl), 394.
4. The remarkable versatility of braille is evident not only in its slow but eventual victory over numerous rival codes, but also in the number and diversity of

languages that continue to use braille transcription. Cf. *World Braille Usage* (Paris: UNESCO; Washington, D.C.: Library of Congress, National Library Service for the Blind and Physically Handicapped, 1990).

5. Catherine Mack, "The Impact of Technology on Braille Literacy," *Journal of Visual Impairment and Blindness* 83 (June 1989): 314.
6. Karen Luxton, Director of the Computer Center for the Visually Impaired, Baruch College, City University of New York, in a personal interview with Tom McNulty, January 31, 1992.
7. Gabriel Farrell, "Avenues of Communication," in *Blindness*, 323.
8. Karen Luxton, interview, *January 31, 1992.*
9. "High Quality of Service Meets Special Needs," *Library of Congress Information Bulletin* 50 (March 25, 1991): 104.
10. "History of the Library of Congress Program," in *That All May Read: Library Service for Blind and Physically Handicapped People* (Washington, D.C.: Library of Congress, National Library Service for the Blind and Physically Handicapped, 1983), 67.
11. Ibid.
12. *FACTS* (Washington, D.C.: Library of Congress, National Library Service for the Blind and Physically Handicapped, January 1991), 1.
13. Vicki Fitzpatrick, "The Sole Source: The Library of Congress National Library Service for the Blind and Physically Handicapped," *Health Libraries Review* 7 (1990): 76.
14. *FACTS*, 1.
15. *Volunteers Who Produce Books: Braille, Tape, Large Print* (Washington, D.C.: Library of Congress, National Library Service for the Blind and Physically Handicapped, 1988), 1.
16. "A History of the National Library Service for Blind and Handicapped Individuals, the Library of Congress," in *That All May Read*, 200.
17. John Wilkinson, Literary Braille Adviser, National Library Service for the Blind and Physically Handicapped, telephone interview with Tom McNulty, March 3, 1992.
18. Claudell S. Stocker, Head, Braille Development Division, National Library Service for the Blind, Library of Congress. "Volunteer Braille Transcribing in the United States," manuscript, n.d., 1.
19. John Wilkinson, interview, March 3, 1992.
20. Ibid.
21. *Projects and Experiments* (Washington D.C.: Library of Congress, National Library Service for the Blind and Physically Handicapped, Summer 1990), 2.
22. Ibid.
23. Ibid., 8.
24. Susan J. Spungin, *Braille Literacy: Issues for Blind Persons, Families, Professionals, and Producers of Braille* (New York: American Foundation for the Blind, n.d), 11.
25. Jane Mandelbaum, interview with Tom McNulty, March 24, 1992.
26. *Projects and Experiments*, 12.
27. Harris, "Inventing Printing for the Blind," 24.
28. James C. Bliss and Mary W. Moore, "The Optacon Reading System," in *The*

Mainstreamed Library: Issues, Ideas, Innovations, edited by Barbara Holland Baskin (Chicago: American Library Assn., 1982), 107.

29. *Library Services for Persons with Disabilities, SPEC Kit 176* (Washington, D.C.: Systems and Procedures Exchange Center, OMS, Association of Research Libraries, July/Aug. 1991), 7.

Chapter Four

Audio Output Systems

Perhaps the most heated debate raging within the blindness community today relates to the use of audio output systems versus the use of braille. The diminished use of braille by a majority of print-impaired individuals has led many blindness professionals to conclude that there is a genuine lack of literacy among members of the community. Proponents of braille believe that reliance upon audio output systems such as the recorded word and synthetic speech devices does not constitute true literacy in the way that the use of tactile systems such as braille does. It is not our intention to enter into this debate. As previously stated, our goal in writing this book has been to describe a variety of methods (tactile, audio, and print-enhanced) that might better integrate all print-impaired individuals into the mainstream reading/research environment.

There are many reasons why braille literacy has declined in recent years. The ability to read and write braille is an acquired skill—it requires training and practice, which takes time and money. Not all print-impaired individuals have had access to the resources that would enable them to acquire this skill. Moreover, since not all print-impaired individuals are completely blind, many have not had the time or inclination to achieve braille literacy. As mentioned in chapter 3, the trend to "mainstream" print-impaired individuals has also reduced their exposure to training in braille. For those with a cognitive learning disability, braille is not normally an asset. Their difficulty is not in recognizing letters printed on a page but rather in processing and comprehending the printed word at a "normal" rate. Since even the most proficient braille readers rarely achieve a so-called normal reading rate, use of the tactile system by learning-disabled individuals would do little to augment their processing speed.

Finally, advances in technology over the past sixty years have greatly increased the level of access to print materials for those who cannot or will not, for whatever reason, learn braille. This chapter will be primarily concerned with these technological advances. But again we wish to reiterate our position that the use of these alternative methods should not be regarded as undermining the need for braille literacy among certain members of the print-impaired community; rather we would assert the need for diversification and flexibility. Surely the individual who is able to read and write braille, make use of audio recordings, and access computer technology by means of one or another adaptive device enjoys a greater degree of independence than does the individual who is strictly confined to any one of these methods. Today, the average print-impaired individual has had at least some contact with each of the access systems named above and it is important that we, as service providers, appreciate the heterogeneity and remarkable ingenuity of the individuals who comprise our target population.

In this chapter we will describe a variety of audio output systems popular today, while remembering that none of these, in and of itself, provides the print-impaired individual with full access to the multitude of literary and reference materials available in most contemporary libraries. Each of the systems described below will have its own purpose and application. From spoken word recordings to electronic text to online database systems, the fully accessible library will offer its print-impaired patrons a wide range of output options.

Our discussion begins with the introduction of talking book technology by the American Foundation for the Blind in the early 1930s and traces the widespread acceptance of this text format within the print-impaired community. There follows a description of "radio reading services," which gained popularity in the 1960s. But it is through an exploration of some surprisingly early research conducted into the development of "reading machines for the blind" that our examination of hi-tech solutions to the problem of access to print is initiated. Although the development of synthetic speech came as a direct result of this early research into reading machines, it was not until the advent of the personal computer in the mid-1980s that the application of this technology was fully exploited to the benefit of the print-impaired individual. It was during this decade of fast-forward technological advance that the proliferation of commercially viable screen-access software designed for use by the print-impaired individual truly began.

Today, the use of computer technology by blind, visually impaired, and learning-disabled individuals is as commonplace as is the use of this technology by the nondisabled population. Indeed, we would submit that the use of computer technology is, in today's information age, even more essential to the educational and economic well-being of the print-impaired adult than to that of the individual for whom the print media present no such obstacles. As our society moves further away from its affinity for paper text formats and closer to the use of electronic texts, the computer literate print-impaired individual will be increasingly able to compete on an equal footing with his or her peers in the workplace, in the classroom, and in ordinary daily activities. This chapter will, therefore, include a discussion of recent projects related to the mass production and dissemination of electronic text formats, some of which were developed with the print-impaired community specifically in mind and others which may benefit them unexpectedly.

Since the nature of today's technology is constantly changing, we will conclude with an examination of current and emerging trends that are likely to have a powerful impact on the print-impaired individual. We will concentrate, predictably, on the growing use of the graphical user interface (GUI) and the problems it generates for the print-impaired computer user who relies predominately on synthetic speech screen-access systems. We will explain the reasons why GUIs pose a threat to current speech technology and describe measures that have been taken to ensure that the speech-dependent computer user not be left behind by advances in technology.

Now that technology has made it possible for the print-impaired individual to access materials that were previously unavailable without the aid of a sighted reader, it is important that the computer industry not lose track of the needs of this community and that service providers such as librarians be well-informed of the range of products that are available. Although we would prefer not to endorse specific products, in this chapter especially it has been impossible to avoid mentioning some of the more popular hard- and software components by name. We have consulted with a number of technology experts and instructors to arrive at the conclusions drawn below. Each of the devices described in the section on synthetic speech access has been independently endorsed by several professionals in the field. For a more complete resource listing, see appendix B.

Spoken Word Recordings

Background

Thomas Edison, in his 1877 patent on the phonograph, included "recorded books for the blind"as a possible application for the new invention, but it was not until 1932 that the American Foundation for the Blind (AFB) began working in earnest on the project.[1] One of the greatest motivational forces behind AFB's development of the talking book was the lack of braille literacy among adults who had been adventitiously blinded. Statistics gathered by the NLS in the 1930s suggested that, "less than twenty percent of the blind population had sufficient skill to make reading library books practicable and less than ten percent sufficient to make it enjoyable."[2] Today, most print-impaired individuals and blindness professionals agree that, for older adults, learning braille is often complicated by a loss of fingertip sensitivity. We would contend that learning the tactile-based reading system is often extremely difficult for anyone who learned to read by visual means. That is, there are psychological factors to be considered as well as loss of tactile sensitivity. As with learning a second language and developing native proficiency, individuals who do not acquire braille reading skills at an early age rarely achieve high levels of proficiency. Thus, many adventitiously blinded individuals never learn to read braille at all.

When AFB began working on the development of the talking book, it was primarily with this older, braille illiterate population in mind. Later, when many veterans of World War II began returning home blinded, paralyzed, or as amputees, the increasing usefulness of talking book technology became even more evident. Not only were the war-injured braille illiterate but many were physically incapable of holding books and turning their pages. Today, our understanding of learning disabilities would further extend the definition of print-impairment to include those individuals who have neither an organic vision loss nor a physical disability but who, because of cognitive impairments, are unable to satisfactorily process the printed word. As stated earlier, braille literacy among these individuals is virtually useless. In fact, for many learning-disabled individuals, auditory reinforcement of the written word is an important learning aid. Thus the need for audio output systems has expanded with our understanding of the nature of learning disabilities.

Indeed, AFB's original target population for talking books was well served by the new medium; statistics collected by NLS in 1938 (just six years after the talking book had first been introduced) indicated that "76% of talking book readers did not read embossed type at all."[3] Given our present, somewhat broader definition of print-impairment, it is not surprising that current statistics would indicate an even greater tendency toward braille illiteracy among talking book users. Again, since the use of audio recordings requires little or no training, it is possible for even the newly print-impaired individual (adventitiously blinded adults, amputees, individuals suffering with progressive neurological diseases, persons recently diagnosed with learning disabilities, etc.) to begin "literary rehabilitation" almost immediately. We use the qualifying adverb "almost" because before print-impaired individuals are able to take advantage of materials produced in braille or on audiocassette, they must first register with the appropriate agencies to obtain the necessary materials and equipment.

Acquisition of Recorded Books

Most of us who have made a trip to any large, contemporary bookstore within the past few years have discovered a fair selection of spoken word cassettes on the shelves.[4] These so-called audio books include titles from diverse fields such as self-help guides, autobiographies read by their authors, and popular fiction. Indeed, listening to tapes has, for many people, presented itself as a pleasant alternative to reading the printed manuscript. These commercial productions, however, bear little resemblance to the materials produced by either the NLS or Recordings for the Blind, Inc. (RFB), and in most cases they do not provide the full range of materials needed by the print-impaired community.

Generally, the recordings available in most bookstores are severely abridged—witness the fact that Dickens' *A Tale of Two Cities* consumes but two sixty-minute cassettes. Since the average individual reads aloud at approximately 150 to 200 words per minute, this would represent roughly 18,000 to 24,000 words or, at best, 50 to 100 pages of written text. On the other hand, the materials produced by NLS and RFB are read in their entirety, and those recorded by the latter group include verbal descriptions of photographs, drawings, maps, charts, and tables as well. Thus, the student who is studying *Hamlet* will, in most cases, be better served by RFB's presentation of the material (replete with preface, commentary, and explanatory footnotes) than by a modern, commercial production which, although narrated by a talented actor and gussied-up with high-quality stereophonic sound effects, does not even contain the full body of the text.

This is not to suggest that the commercial recordings do not often benefit the print-impaired public enormously. There is generally a fairly substantial lag time before a contemporary bestseller is recorded by NLS and often certain works never manage to make it into the NLS or RFB collection at all. Moreover, in the case of an autobiography or some other work read aloud by its author, there might be a genuine advantage to obtaining the commercial recording. Finally, the commercial recordings are, of course, purchased, whereas the materials distributed by both NLS and RFB are merely on loan to the subscriber. Thus, we would urge those in charge of library acquisitions not to automatically exclude the commercial recordings.

While the commercial recordings are readily obtainable and would certainly demonstrate a good-faith effort on the library's behalf to serve its print-impaired patrons, the acquisition of these materials should in no way replace the use of the two nationally-known, government-sanctioned library services for the print-impaired individual who has been formally certified (see chapter 3 for eligibility requirements). Both the NLS and RFB have had a longtime commitment to the print-impaired public and they serve their members well.

Origins of the NLS and RFB

The National Library Service for the Blind and Physically Handicapped was formally established as a division of the Library of Congress in 1931 after the passage of the Pratt-Smoot Bill, which allowed Congress to appropriate funds for the production and dissemination of braille texts.[5] In 1935, just three short years after the introduction of the talking book, Congress appropriated increased funds to the project to cover the production of the recorded texts which, as previously mentioned, had gained immediate popularity among print-impaired readers. The increased funds were necessary because the recorded books were not only more expensive to produce than was braille but also because their use required access to special playback equipment. Since the purchase of this equipment would have represented a financial hardship for many of the library's patrons, it was eventually decided that the library itself should retain ownership of the playback machines, which would then be loaned to qualified users. The period of the loan was unspecified; it was simply agreed that the equipment would be returned to the library once the print-impaired user could no longer make use of it.

During the late 1940s, the number of war-blind who were returning to college under the GI Bill contributed greatly to the growing need for college textbooks in accessible format. As few of the war-blind were fully (or even partially) braille literate, recorded books were generally the preferred medium. During 1947 and 1948, numerous volunteer recording groups cropped up throughout the United States to meet the academic and vocational rehabilitation needs of this population. As there was no real quality control or enforceable code of standards among these disparate volunteer groups, RFB was established by Anne MacDonald to coordinate and oversee the development of a national volunteer network.

Today, these two library services produce most of the materials for the print-impaired. As mentioned earlier, there are a number of commercial firms that produce and distribute spoken word recordings, but as their intended audience is not specifically print-impaired, these recordings do not always meet the special needs of these individuals. It should be further noted that there are a number of other organizations (both volunteer and profit-making) that produce materials designed for a print-impaired readership. But these groups often represent special-interest groups and do not try to meet the academic and literary needs of the entire print-impaired population.[6] The differences between NLS and RFB are noteworthy and will be discussed in the section titled "Text Formats and Quality Control."

Eligibility Requirements

Because authors of books produced in either braille or recorded format do not receive royalty compensation for these texts, both NLS and RFB require their patrons to submit some type of eligibility certification. That is, the special copyright agreements held by both library services demand that measures be taken to ensure that only qualified individuals be permitted to use the audio recordings they produce. Generally speaking, qualification depends on a person's having a physical impairment that prevents him or her from reading an ordinary printed page. In the case of an individual who is visually, physically, or neurologically impaired, both NLS and RFB will accept verification of this condition from a physician, blindness professional, or some other service provider, including teachers and librarians. Eligibility certification for both agencies becomes slightly more complex when dealing with individuals having a learning disability. In fact, the two agencies differ considerably in their approach to this type of print-impairment. NLS will certify a learning-disabled individual's eligibility if and only if verification of a physically-based condition is received from a medical doctor. RFB, on the other hand, will accept authorization from no one but a recognized learning disability specialist.

Libraries may register for institutional membership with either or both of the two agencies. In this way, materials may be acquired on loan and made available for use by eligible patrons. Both RFB and NLS produce print catalogs of their publications. Librarians having access to BRS/BLND may search the online database for the availability of texts in recorded format.[7] To register with NLS or RFB, contact the cooperating regional library in your area. It should be emphasized that the recordings produced by both agencies require the use of specially adapted playback equipment. Like the recordings themselves, this equipment is also available on loan to qualified individuals and institutions through the NLS. The American Printing House for the Blind in Louisville, Kentucky, also manufactures and sells equipment that will play NLS talking books and RFB audiocassettes. RFB does not, however, deal in the distribution of playback equipment.

Production

It is perhaps easy to understand why NLS became involved in the distribution of playback equipment during the 1930s when audio technology was in its infancy and owning a phonograph of one's own was quite extravagant. Today the need to acquire audio equipment from an agency such as the NLS is perplexing. However, as might be expected, the materials recorded by both NLS and RFB are formatted differently from standard commercial recordings. NLS produces both audiocassettes and flexible disk recordings. The latter, which only slightly resemble commercial disk recordings (LP albums and 45s), are played at a speed of eight revolutions per minute (rpm), while the cassettes produced by both NLS and RFB (as well as those produced by many other independent agencies dealing specifically with recordings for the blind) play at a speed of 15/16 inches per second (ips). In contrast, standard albums play at 33 rpm, singles at 45 rpm. Therefore it is unlikely that any commercial turntable would be able to play NLS flexible disks properly. Commercial audiocassettes are generally recorded on two tracks (stereo) and play at a speed of 1 7/8 ips. Not only are NLS and RFB texts recorded at a slower speed but they are produced in a monophonic four-track format. Again, the average cassette deck or walkman is incapable of handling this special format properly.

The reasons for the divergent formats are at least twofold. Clearly, the slower speeds allow more information to be stored on each unit. Additionally, the use of the four-track format on the cassettes further augments the amount of material that can be stored on each tape. The reader is reminded of our Dickens example: the NLS recording of *A Tale of Two Cities* consumes three cassettes recorded on four tracks and at 15/16 ips. Imagine how many cassettes this book would require and how much more cumbersome and expensive it would be if recorded at double the speed and with half as much space per tape. Although the postal laws were amended in 1934 to permit the free mailing of recorded books for the blind, the financial burden of purchasing enough tapes to record some of the world's great literature might be prohibitive.

The second, less obvious (but surely more interesting and important) reason why the audio recordings are produced in nonstandard formats involves the nature of the copyright agreement between NLS, RFB, and the publishers. Indeed, the copyright permission that is so freely granted these two library services is virtually dependent upon the fact that the materials are produced in nonstandard formats and therefore require the use of specially adapted playback equipment. Since individuals wishing to borrow equipment from NLS must certify their eligibility to receive service from the agency, publishers who might otherwise fear the loss of royalty compensation can be relatively certain that only individuals for whom the print copies of their texts are useless will take advantage of the recorded books. Why are the publishers so concerned about profit loss? As Susan Mosakowski, director of the talking book recording studio at the New York Regional Library for the Blind, points out, there has been an increased number of inquiries from the general population in recent years. She explains that passersby who understand that the library lends books in recorded format will often come in and attempt to borrow recordings. "There's a cultural move toward immediacy. We're talking about reading in general. We're seeing an increase in fast material," Mosakowski asserts.[8] While true bibliophiles may object to this trend, we can certainly anticipate its having a beneficial effect upon the print-impaired population. The ability to walk into a local bookstore and purchase an accessible copy of a popular novel, abridged or not, can do much to elevate the print-impaired consumer's involvement in mainstream society.

Text Formats and Quality Control

As described in chapter 3, advances made in technology during recent years have made the in-house production of braille materials readily achievable in many cases. With the help of a standard PC, braille printer, and Duxbury translation software, original source documents are easily produced in braille format. Add an optical character recognition device to the configuration and a wide range of print materials may be quickly and easily converted. The in-house production of audio recordings, while less technologically complex, is perhaps impractical and, in many instances, may prove unnecessary. The librarian who seeks to provide a print-impaired patron with access to one or another text in audio format is advised to verify first (either through a BLND search or by contacting NLS and RFB directly) that the text is not already available. The NLS' current collection comprises fifty-nine thousand titles, and the number increases by approximately two thousand per year. For the student, a search of RFB's collection of academic and scholarly works will generally yield a positive result. Most popular high school and college textbooks are already available from this library in recorded format and those that are not may be requested. RFB, unlike NLS, will generally produce recordings for any of its registered borrowers on demand.

The production of audio recordings is strictly monitored by these two agencies—both adhere to high standards of quality control, and it is unlikely that individuals wishing to produce independent recordings would be able to claim the degree of accuracy and quality NLS and RFB maintain. We would, however, suggest that libraries publishing monthly newsletters or information packets make an effort to produce audio copies of this material in-house. Print-impaired patrons need this type of material in order to participate fully in library services and activities, and in most cases it is easiest for the library to produce them itself. Regarding the production of full-length texts, however, the job is better left to the experts. Moreover, both NLS and RFB maintain copyright agreements with a variety of publishing firms, whereas procuring such permission might be difficult for an independent facility.

As mentioned earlier, both NLS and RFB use a nonstandard recording format for their audio recordings so as to conserve tape and verify that only qualified individuals have physical access to them. The playback equipment available on loan from NLS is just that—playback equipment—it has no recording capability. The machines sold by APH, on the other hand, do have four-track, 15/16 ips recording capabilities. However, it is perhaps inadvisable for independent libraries to produce their information bulletins, etc., in this special format, since guaranteeing that all potential patrons have access to the playback equipment is impossible. Many older, visually impaired adults, for example, may not be registered with either of the two agencies. Most individuals do, nonetheless, have access to standard playback equipment, so it would be wisest to use that for library bulletins and announcements. The librarian can, however, play an important role in making the print-impaired individual aware of the services provided by

NLS and RFB, and may help qualified patrons register for these services (see the section on Eligibility Requirements above).

Audiophiles will recognize that dividing a cassette tape into four tracks and then recording the information at half the usual speed will seriously degrade the sound quality of the recording. This degeneration of sound quality would be an issue were the recordings attempting to reproduce the beauty and elegance of a Mozart symphony. Since, however, we are dealing with the spoken word, the question of sound degradation does not come into play in the same way it would with music. Remember that the primary purpose of the talking books has never been to provide the print-impaired individual with an outstanding performance of one or another literary text; instead, the fundamental objective has been to provide access to materials that would be otherwise inaccessible. Nonetheless, the recordings engineered and produced by both NLS and RFB are made in special recording studios using state-of-the-art equipment. In most cases, the texts are read by highly qualified professionals. In fact, NLS relies almost exclusively on theatrically trained actors to produce its talking books.

The recording process is involved, requiring three individuals per project: a narrator who actually records the text, a monitor who is present throughout each of the recording sessions to verify that the narrator does not inadvertently skip over text or mispronounce words, and finally a reviewer who checks the finished product for errors that might have been missed by both narrator and monitor. Not everyone is qualified to narrate a talking book for the NLS; even the regional libraries, which rely on volunteer narrators, adhere to the National Library Service's high standards. As Susan Mosakowski explains, potential narrators often have the wrong idea about their role in the process—they can become overzealous and lapse into strange accents, unusual voice qualities, or other affectations. "As a reader of these books, you want to have space for yourself. The narrator has to be somewhat transparent," Mosakowski asserts.[9]

RFB's approach is slightly different from that of the NLS and this is perhaps a result of the disparity between the types of materials recorded by both services. RFB deals exclusively in academic and vocational texts while NLS does not. The materials produced by RFB are directly aimed at students. Their narrators, therefore, are obliged to describe charts, maps, photographs, drawings, and diagrams on a regular basis. Since students must have the ability to cite research materials properly, all pagination and pertinent bibliographic data are recorded along with the body of the text. Although RFB relies solely on the service of volunteer narrators, efforts are made to ensure that only qualified readers record its texts. Indeed, an individual narrating a computer science, calculus, or biology textbook must be familiar enough with the discipline to interpret scientific or mathematical notation and any related charts or figures without faltering. Thus, volunteer or not, RFB's narrators must adhere to that organization's high standards.

Many of RFB's studios specialize in one or another particular discipline. In some cases this is by design; in others the specialization has been a natural outgrowth of the demographics of the region. As Laurie Facciarossa, public information officer at RFB, explains, both the Philadelphia and Boston studios have been designated as science and technology-based units, whereas others have simply "carved their own niche. The New York studio is recognized as being strong in art and art history. Washington tends to have a lot of people who have been in the diplomatic corp or other types of foreign service, so they have a lot of expertise in foreign languages."[10] Both RFB and NLS perform their tasks quite well, together serving the multifaceted needs of the print-impaired public.

Readers, Reading Services, and Reading Machines

Prior to AFB's introduction of the spoken word recording, print-impaired individuals who were not braille literate had only one option for accessing print material: the use of a sighted reader. Self-determination and independence have been longtime goals of this group, however, and the use of sighted readers is essentially antithetical to achieving these goals. As we have seen, the use of braille and audio recordings has done much to further the independence of the print-impaired individual, but there is a broad range of materials that do not lend themselves well to production in either of these formats. Newspapers, magazines, reference books, and telephone directories are all examples of the type of material not easily formatted in braille or on audiocassette. Newspapers and magazines are basically ephemeral; they would lose their timely nature if reproduced in braille or audio format, given the time needed to transcribe them. Braille versions of reference books or telephone directories are cumbersome; searching through such texts on audiocassette is extremely difficult because of the sequential nature of the medium. For many people, using a sighted reader is still the most effective manner of accessing "disposable" information. But reliance on a sighted assistant is no longer necessary, for technology has advanced to the point where it is now possible for the print-impaired reader to independently scan a variety of printed materials using only mechanical and electronic aids. Most print-impaired individuals would agree that the ability to look up phone numbers oneself, conduct research independently, or even browse in a leisurely fashion through the latest issue of a popular magazine is preferable to working with an assistant. In this section we will first look at the advent of reading programs and reading machines, and then discuss the breakthrough achieved by optical character recognition, synthetic speech, and screen-access software.

Radio Reading Services

The need to supplement materials produced in accessible formats was recognized as early as 1897, when the Library of Congress established a program for its blind patrons that included "oral readings each day, a weekly recital, art gallery visits, garden parties, dramatic entertainments, river excursions and teas."[11] Shortly thereafter, similar programs followed in Cincinnati and San Francisco. But it was not until the late 1960s that the first radio reading services were created to provide the print-impaired public with access to newspapers and periodicals.[12] Radio reading services, as the name implies, take advantage of broadcast frequencies to transmit information over the air. The services use a subcarrier channel of the standard broadcast band and, again, can only be accessed with the help of specially adapted equipment. While these services do provide the print-impaired individual with increased access to news, they cannot offer the user true independence. Radio reading announcers are tied to a strict schedule and must often condense the texts they are reading, so that once more we are dealing with only partial access to the print copy. While this is not truly an issue of censorship, it does impinge upon the print-impaired individual's freedom of choice. He or she is confined to reading the abridged materials at the scheduled time, in the designated order, with no ability to skip those stories that are of no interest. Moreover, there is no way of saving the material for later reference or review.

In 1987, an automated telephone reading service was established in Flint, Michigan, to provide print-impaired readers with greater access to news. The service, called "Newspapers for the Blind," operates in the same way as any automated phone service: using a touchtone keypad, the user selects the stories whose headlines interest him. Both New Mexico and Minnesota maintain similar daily news services. While the nature of the telephone service affords the user a greater degree of choice, there is still no easy way of storing the information for reference or review. This problem has been resolved in Sweden, where a radio reading service broadcasts its news over an FM band overnight to the homes of print-impaired subscribers, where the data are then stored in electronic format. The subscriber can then review the information using a home computer and a screen-access device the following morning. This solution, however, presupposes access to the necessary technology. Indeed, it is primarily through access to technology that print-impaired readers will find their greatest independence.

Reading Machines

Franklin S. Cooper, in a 1950 essay on research trends in the development of "reading machines for the blind," asserts "there is evident need for some device which will allow him to read for himself the wide range of materials available in print but not in braille or on records. A reading machine capable of producing intelligible sounds from the printed page of the average book, magazine or typewritten page would go far towards fulfilling this requirement. Such a device can hardly be expected to cope with illustrations or with symbols and formulae and it thus appears that an auxiliary capable of producing relief images is also needed."[13] Today, both such devices exist and not only do many print-impaired individuals have access to optical character recognition equipment and braille embossers at their local libraries but many individuals own such equipment themselves. It is highly unlikely that Cooper or any of his colleagues in the acoustical sciences would have predicted the level of complexity and sophistication this equipment would achieve in recent decades. But it is largely due to the research conducted by linguists and acoustical engineers at the Haskins Laboratory in the mid-1940s that today print-impaired readers are able to independently access an enormous variety of print materials.

Historical Development

According to Cooper's essay, it was Willoughby Smith's 1873 discovery that selenium was influenced by light that led to Alexander Graham Bell's invention of the photophone three years later.[14] The photophone was a device that was able to transmit sound on a beam of light. Bell's work enabled Foe d'Albe to develop an implement called the "exploring optaphone," which was used to help visually impaired individuals detect open doors and windows. This invention, in turn, led to Barr and Stroud's perfection of the "reading optaphone" in 1918. Although special photophonic books had been produced as early as 1902, the reading optaphone represents the first successful mechanically-based audio translation of ordinary print.

The reading optaphone did not, however, translate text to speech; rather, it produced a series of musical tones corresponding to the configuration of black and white images on the printed page. It was extremely difficult to learn and reports indicate that even the most proficient students rarely attained reading rates higher than thirty or forty words per minute. Remember that the average individual reads aloud at a rate of 150 to 200 words per minute; he reads silently at an even faster speed. Thus, while the goal of the reading optaphone was commendable, limitations in the technology of the day severely limited its application. Fortunately, researchers did not abandon their goal, and eventually work done by both RCA and Haskins led to the development of a recognition device that could not only recognize printed letters on a page but could then reproduce them in the sounds of English. With Haskins' development of the sound spectrograph and the pattern playback, both optical character recognition and synthetic speech were born.

Optical Character Recognition and Kurzweil Computer Products

Most print-impairment specialists and librarians have by now had a fair bit of exposure to one or another of Raymond Kurzweil's text-to-speech optical character recognition devices as both the early Kurzweil Reading Machine (KRM) and the newer Kurzweil Personal Reader (KPR) are in widespread use in hundreds of public facilities throughout the country. Indeed, there remain few print-impaired individuals who have not received some degree of training with one of these devices. The prototype of Kurzweil's reading machine was available in 1974. Three years later, the device was being distributed to consumers and by the early 1980s, most large libraries and academic institutions had obtained the equipment. By today's standards, the original KRM is too large, slow, and inaccurate to be useful. A dinosaur by comparison to the sleek, new Kurzweil Personal Reader with its speed, interface capabilities, and accuracy, the original KRM nevertheless served its users well.

Although optical character recognition had been more or less commonly in use since the 1960s, Kurzweil's product was revolutionary in its approach. OCR technology had already been used to decipher "black numerals on the bottoms of checks and pricing and inventory control stripes on packages in the grocery store . . . those numerals and stripes have to be very precisely and consistently formed, however, in order to be legible to the computer."[15] Never before had an electronic device been capable of recognizing such a wide array of fonts, matching the recognized patterns to those stored in its internal memory, and then synthesizing the result to produce comprehensible speech. Again, by today's standards, neither the speech quality nor the accuracy of the original KRM would be considered particularly sophisticated, but in the pre-PC era of the early 1980s this technology represented unprecedented independence for the print-impaired reader. For the first time, one could independently access print materials of choice literally with the push of a button.

Despite the fact that the new technology could offer the print-impaired user an unmatched degree of independence, studies indicate that those early machines were severely underutilized.[16] As the researchers at Haskins had suspected, a successful reading machine would have to concentrate on simplicity of operation—it would not make unreasonable demands on its users. The earlier reading optaphone had, in many regards, been a brilliant example of electrical engineering; it failed primarily because its users could neither master nor forgive its complexity. And although the original KRM had made enormous technological advances, its operation was not entirely intuitive. Users required fairly extensive training, the strange sing-song quality of its speech patterns posed difficulties for many users, and its accuracy, though without electronic precedent, still did not equal that of a live reader.

The Kurzweil Personal Reader, which made its debut in 1989, is considerably easier to master. It is far more compact than was the old model; its keypad has fewer buttons and their functions are presented in a somewhat more intuitive manner. Moreover, the new device incorporates the use of an extremely sophisticated speech synthesizer (the DECTalk by Digital Equipment Corporation) so that even the naive listener is impressed by its voice quality, finding it immediately comprehensible. The machine's accuracy, though not entirely infallible, is vastly improved. Moreover, it now has the ability to inform its users of an unrecognized character and the presence of a photograph or page that is either upside down or "too difficult" to be interpreted accurately. Kurzweil trainers report that not only do today's users adapt more readily to the concepts involved in the equipment's operation but that the new KPRs are being used with far greater frequency than were the original systems.

Optical character recognition technology has advanced by such leaps and bounds in recent years that today there are a number of comparable systems that compete with Kurzweil's product for a place in the print-impaired market. Adhoc Reading Systems, Telesensory, and Personal Data Systems, Inc., manufacture and distribute OCR equipment that performs as well as does the KPR. These systems are not, however, stand-alone units as is the KPR, but must be interfaced with a PC that has been outfitted with a text-editor and adaptive equipment that enables the print-impaired user to access the screen.[17]

Technological Advancements and Synthetic Speech

Many of the researchers who worked on Haskins' original reading machine project were not only well-versed in acoustical and electrical engineering but in linguistics and the behavioral sciences as well. They therefore possessed a collective understanding of the human limitations that might affect their project's progress. Most of us are familiar with the popular acronym KISS (Keep It Simple, Stupid) used in the computer sciences to warn programmers against developing systems that are too complex for the average individual to operate independently. Many of those early Kurzweil trainers learned firsthand of this caveat's meaning when confronted with the perplexing underutilization of the original KRM. Although the equipment could provide its users with an extraordinary degree of access to previously unavailable materials, the print-impaired user was, in the late 1970s and early 1980s, not computer savvy enough to adjust to the equipment's demands. Today, with computers in common use across the country and frequently already in the homes of visually impaired, blind, and learning-disabled individuals, learning to operate even the most complex computer equipment is far less of a problem. Technological advancements made during the past five years in particular have, for the most part, allowed the print-impaired individual to keep in step with the mainstream computer user. And it has, in many respects, been as a direct result of this technological progress that the print-impaired individual has gained independent access to a broader range of print materials than ever before.

Synthetic Speech and Screen-Access Software

The ability to use a PC keyboard and its video display relies, for many print-impaired individuals, on synthetic speech technology. This technology is composed of two main components: a speech synthesizer and accompanying screen-access software. The synthesizer is a hardware device that may be either an external peripheral unit or an internal card. It is the synthesizer that produces the actual sounds, which are generally channeled through a small, external speaker. The screen-access software is, as its name suggests, a program that interprets the data that are sent to the video display. This software is memory resident, which means that once it has been loaded into memory, it remains there until the computer is rebooted. Although the screen-access program is resident in the computer's memory at all times, it is entirely transparent to any applications software that may be running. In this way, the print-impaired user may interact with word processors, database systems, spreadsheet management programs, telecommunications packages, and the like in virtually the same way a sighted computer user does.

Screen-access software is specifically designed not to interfere with the functions of applications software. Occasionally, applications functions will interfere with the standard configuration of the screen-access software but the more sophisticated packages allow their users to bypass or override applications functions that might cause conflicts with the adaptive device. Unfortunately, no speech-based screen-access system is yet fully able to interpret graphic images, so that access to computers that rely upon a graphical user interface is still extremely limited. We will address this issue shortly. At present, the vast majority of synthetic speech screen-access programs are designed to work with character-based computers such as the IBM PC and compatible systems. The way in which the character-based computers transmit data to the video display is ideally suited to the use of synthetic speech; in any case, it presents software developers with no particular difficulties. Since the information that is to be sent to the screen is stored in ASCII format in a text buffer, the screen-access software may simply look to this buffer for the data it needs. After the data have been procured in ASCII format, they can be channeled through the synthesizer to the external speaker. The result is generally a highly-comprehensible (if somewhat robotic) audio representation of the sounds of English—or whatever language the program and synthesizer have been designed to interpret.

Growth and Development

As previously discussed, the development of modern synthetic speech technology has its genesis in research conducted at the Haskins Laboratory in the 1940s. It was not, however, until the mid-1980s that use of synthetic speech screen-access systems became relatively common among print-impaired individuals. Kurzweil's reading machine, of course, relied upon a speech synthesizer and proprietary software to produce a verbal representation of the scanned material, but it was the widespread introduction of the personal computer that allowed the development of several commercially viable synthetic speech screen-review software packages.

Myrna Votta, an adaptive technology specialist and instructor with the New York Association for the Blind, recalls that prior to 1986 there were but two or three speech-based screen-access software packages available for use by blind and visually impaired computer users. She explains, however, that, by the end of that year, the development of such systems began, "fast and furious."[18] Today, the synthetic speech screen-access software market is highly competitive and the visually impaired computer user is presented with a number of options when selecting an adaptive device for personal use. Institutions seeking to purchase synthetic speech equipment should be aware of not only the variety of choices currently available but of some appropriate selection criteria as well. Below, we will outline these criteria in relation to six of today's most popular packages: Business Vision by Artic Technologies, Flipper by Omnichron, JAWS by Henter-Joyce, Screen-Reader by IBM, Softvert by Telesensory Systems, and Vocal-eyes by GW Micro.[19]

With the exception of Vocal-eyes, which is a relatively new product, each of the six software packages in the above list has demonstrated a remarkable ability to endure the rigors of an industry where change is a key factor in determining success. The very nature of screen-access technology demands that developers keep up with changes made in standard applications software. There must be a constant effort to maintain access to commercial business applications as well as to improve upon current access techniques. While it is not our intention to endorse any one screen-access system in particular, it must be noted that the packages we have elected to evaluate have, by their longevity, indicated considerable commercial viability. Our inclusion of Vocal-eyes, though new to the market, is based upon this product's quality and immediate popularity.

Selection Criteria

While it is impossible to endorse one screen-access system over another, there are several important issues to be aware of and features to look for when selecting a synthetic speech system for use in an institutional setting. We define these selection criteria as follows: compatibility, memory management, documentation and technical support, functionality, and ease of use. Below we will discuss each of these criteria with specific reference to the software packages named in the preceding section. Indeed, each of the six systems we have identified meet the minimal requirements of our independent selection criteria. Again, this is not to suggest that other programs do not meet our criteria as well, but rather that these six exemplify the standards one would hope to uphold when purchasing adaptive equipment.

Compatibility

With the exception of a package called OutSpoken (discussed below), there are currently no commercially available synthetic speech screen-access programs that work with graphics-based computer systems such as the Apple Macintosh. The present discussion will, therefore, focus entirely on IBM and compatible systems. Generally speaking, most synthetic speech screen-review programs will run with any MS-DOS-based computer, but users having questions about hardware compatibility are encouraged to contact the screen-access software manufacturer directly. Hardware specifications become increasingly significant in this age of PS/2s, laptop, and notebook computers. Indeed, IBM's Screen-Reader was specifically designed for use with the PS/2 line of computers, and although it is compatible with earlier versions of the PC, an additional interface card is required.

Remember that speech-based screen-access systems rely upon the use of a synthesizer. It is therefore imperative to verify that the synthesizer you select is not only supported by the screen-access software you intend to install but also compatible with your hardware configuration. For example, until recently, Artic Technologies was the only company manufacturing internal speech cards that were compatible with laptop computers and the PS/2 microchannel architecture. Since the purpose of a laptop is portability, one would not want to be dependent upon a cumbersome external synthesizer. Thus, prior to Aicom's development of the internal Accent synthesizer for the PS/2 laptop, one would have had to purchase an Artic Synphonix synthesizer for use with a laptop. While using the Artic card does not mandate use of the Artic software, using an Artic card with software other than Artic Business Vision does require the installation of a special program called Sonixtts, which is only available from Artic Technologies. Moreover, the Artic card is "married" to its software; each card is sold with a specific, serial-numbered Artic Business Vision or Sonixtts program, and the card will not function without its proper software companion.

Fortunately, most screen-access software manufacturers are explicit in describing system requirements, synthesizer support, and hardware compatibility. Thus, before purchasing a synthesizer, it is advisable to consult with the screen-access software manufacturer. For those who wish to purchase additional programs to work with synthesizers that have been previously procured, it will be equally important to verify software compatibility. Unfortunately, not all screen-access systems support all synthesizer types, although few are as proprietary in their approach as Artic. While many screen-access systems have been designed to work best with one or another synthesizer (usually the device manufactured and/or distributed by the software development company itself), most programs do offer the end user a variety of options. But again, it is important to be keenly aware of individual hardware configurations that may affect compatibility as well. As previously mentioned, the PS/2 microchannel architecture will impose limitations on one's array of choices, as does this system's lack of expansion slots. Indeed, the size and number of internal expansion slots will be crucial in determining synthesizer compatibility. External synthesizers tend to impose fewer hardware constraints but they are often more expensive and considerably more bulky than internal cards. They do, however, completely circumnavigate the potentially problematic microchannel architecture.

An equally important compatibility issue relates not to hardware configurations but to applications software. When selecting a particular screen-access system, it will be necessary to verify that the program is, in fact, fully compatible with each of the commercial applications users will need to access. It would be unusual, indeed, to discover software conflicts between a screen-access system and programs such as WordPerfect, dBase, or Lotus 1-2-3. Most screen-access programs have been designed with at least these three popular applications in mind. In fact, many of the packages we evaluated (including JAWS, Screen-Reader, Softvert and Vocal-eyes) supply users with predefined configuration files that can be automatically loaded with one or another application. These configurations (JAWS and Artic refer to the customization files as *configurations*, whereas they are called *profiles* by Screen-Reader, *environments* by Softvert, and *sets* by Vocal-eyes) provide the screen-access software with instructions for monitoring important portions of the screen, following lightbars, interpreting cursor position, etc. For example, a WP.Set file in Vocal-eyes monitors the Word-Perfect status line, automatically informing users of any pertinent change (e.g., when the Insert key is pressed and the user enters overwrite mode, the word "typeover" is verbalized). A Softvert 123.VU file will help users interpret cursor position relative to cell addresses, read the menu bar that appears on line two, and voice highlighted choices. The configuration files are designed to provide the visually impaired user with easy access to important program-specific functions.

Designing one's own configuration files is generally quite easy for the advanced user but packages that are equipped with a series of predefined configurations can be extremely helpful to new users. Indeed, IBM's Screen-Reader offers its users a high-level programming language (called the Profile Access Language or PAL) with which to design complex configuration files. The advantage to PAL is, naturally, its power and sophistication. This power and sophistication has enabled Screen-Reader users to write profiles for programs as diverse as DisplayWrite, MicroSoft Works, DOS versions 3.3 through 5, 3270 and 5250 terminal emulation, Q&A, and ProComm Plus. Since writing profiles under PAL is often difficult for even the most experienced users, IBM regularly distributes new profiles to its registered Screen-Reader users.

Institutions that wish to provide users with access to a broad range of applications software should investigate issues concerning both the availability of predefined configurations and the ease with which individual users may create their own configurations. The question of user-defined configurations may be of utmost importance to libraries that wish to provide their print-impaired patrons with access to online database and card catalog systems.

Memory Management

Screen-access systems, whether they produce audio, tactile, or large print output, are known as TSR programs. The letters TSR stand for "terminate and stay resident." As previously explained, this means that the access software is loaded into the computer's memory and remains there until the system is rebooted. The adaptive TSR will, therefore, consume some amount of random access memory (RAM). Fortunately, most screen-access systems are designed to use very little memory. For example, both Vocaleyes and Flipper require considerably less than 60K of RAM whereas Artic/Business Vision and Softvert require slightly more at approximately 70 to 80K. Screen-Reader and JAWS operate best with 128K of available RAM. These memory consumption figures can, however, be reduced by loading the adaptive TSR into extended (XMS) or expanded (EMS) memory. Loading the screen-access program into the upper memory area or loading it "high" is desirable when applications software require a great deal of RAM. Moreover, if more than one TSR is running (e.g., network shells, packages such as SideKick, or screen-enlarging software), it will be extremely important to minimize RAM consumption wherever possible. Remember, too, that the amount of memory used by the screen-access program will be slightly increased with each configuration, profile, environment, or set file that is loaded, and will vary according to the complexity of these files. If the screen-access software allows users to load supplemental key label and/or character dictionaries, even more memory will be used by the adaptive TSR.

Loading a program high requires the use of a memory manager such as QRAM (for 80286 machines) or QEMM (for 80386 machines) from QuarterDeck. QuarterDeck's products have been tested for use with screen-access software by developers at Artic Technologies, Henter-Joyce, and GW Micro. Developers also report success using "386 To The Max."

Additionally, MS-DOS 5 is equipped with device drivers (HIMEM.SYS and EMM386.EXE) that will enable the use of either extended or expanded memory or both.[20] PCs that use either the 8088 or 8086 CPU have no XMS abilities, so that loading a program high on these systems requires the use of expanded memory. Using expanded memory tends to be somewhat trickier than using extended memory, so wherever possible, using extended memory is preferable. If, however, a system does not have XMS capabilities, it is generally worth the trouble of attempting to use the EMS since, in the case of a program such as Vocal-eyes, for example, DOS RAM consumption will be reduced from 60K to 4K.

Documentation and Technical Support

Most readers who have had occasion to purchase computer equipment or software will immediately realize the need for comprehensive product documentation. New users will rely primarily upon the documentation to install, learn, and become proficient with their screen-access systems. This documentation must, therefore, be easy to understand, logically arranged, and provided in an accessible format. Each of the packages we reviewed does provide their users with documentation on disk, in print, and on audiocassette. Perhaps because of the cost of producing braille, few screen-access software manufacturers furnish users with documentation in this format. Of the packages we examined, only Flipper offered its users a braille copy of the complete documentation; Softvert does come with a command summary in braille. And both Artic and Screen-Reader will supply users with a braille copy of the documentation at an additional cost.

While having a machine-readable version of a screen-access program's documentation can be extremely helpful to the advanced user, audio recordings or braille documentation generally prove more useful to the new user. Without a screen-access program already loaded into memory, text files describing installation procedures and introductory access techniques are virtually useless to the visually impaired user. Thus, products that offer their users training tapes and online tutorials can be preferable to those that do not. Indeed, JAWS, Screen-Reader, and Vocal-eyes score several points in this area. Each of these three provide users with clear and complete documentation, but it is IBM's Screen-Reader that must be singled out for commentary.

While the audiocassettes supplied with JAWS and Vocal-eyes help new users through step-by-step operating instructions, the Screen-Reader package takes a two-pronged approach to its tutorials that is quite effective. Screen-Reader uses both an audio recording and online tutorial to teach new users how to operate the system. This approach is similar to that employed by commercial firms such as Fliptrack. The online tutorials do not permit users to "get ahead of themselves." If a user attempts to access a Screen-Reader function that has not yet been introduced, an error message is encountered. In this way, new users cannot get lost or confused since it is absolutely impossible to access advanced features until they have been fully explained. Additionally, the Screen-Reader package includes a set of online reference books that can be read using specially designed profiles. In this way, new users need not be familiar with either a word processor or the DOS TYPE command in order to immediately access electronic documentation files.

Both Flipper and Softvert offer their users friendly alternatives to the DOS TYPE command as well. Flipper includes a program called Look, which when used in conjunction with the *index* file, allows the user to conduct an online subject search. Read.com, distributed with the Softvert software, is unlike the DOS TYPE command in that it permits users to scroll forward and backward through ASCII text files as well as search for particular text strings. But, again, new users who have limited proficiency with screen navigation techniques may find the use of documentation files considerably more frustrating than listening to cassette tutorials. Fortunately, each of the six programs we have been discussing includes an online help facility, and once users have gained some familiarity with the screen-access system, using the help facility can be quite effective. Indeed, Artic's online help is remarkably comprehensive and easy to access. To its credit as well, Artic is the only package that includes a program to assist new users in learning the standard 101 keyboard.

With the possible exception of JAWS and Vocal-eyes, most of the documentation we evaluated was sorely lacking in detail regarding advanced program features. Both the Artic and Vert manuals tend to gloss over important program functions that might enable experienced users to maximize efficiency, and IBM's discussion of the Profile Access Language is truly inadequate, although the company does issue a quarterly newsletter to keep users up-to-date with new profiles and Screen-Reader developments. In any case, the ability to obtain technical support from the software developers directly as well as from other users will be essential. Naturally, all six of the manufacturers whose products we reviewed provide registered users with telephone support. Artic, Henter-Joyce, IBM, and TSI maintain toll-free technical support hotlines. Unfortunately, it is often the case that the individuals who man the technical support lines do not have true firsthand experience with the screen-access program. While they may be perfectly competent technicians, they are not always end users themselves. It is for this reason that we would encourage user networking. AFB maintains a national database of adaptive technology specialists, consultants, and users for the purpose of providing individuals and institutions with access to community-based technical support.

Myrna Votta raises an interesting issue regarding the availability of community-based support: "I think each area of the country has its own regional program. In the south it's JAWS because Henter-Joyce is headquartered in Florida. California is Flipper because Omnichron is in Berkeley. New York, New Jersey, and Connecticut lean toward Artic, Vert, and now Vocaleyes."[21] Thus, when purchasing screen-access equipment, it may be advisable to consider the geographic area's "program of preference." In the final analysis, individual end users may be of greatest assistance to one another where adaptive technology is concerned. As Jay Leventhal of AFB's National Technology Center points out, often potential users of one or another adaptive device will want to engage in a frank discussion of a program's particular pros and cons and require demonstrations of system features or information not included in product literature. He asserts that such discussions and demonstrations should take place "not in front of a salesman" but with private users of the equipment itself.[22]

Functionality

As with most off-the-shelf word processing, database, and spreadsheet management software, the vast majority of popular synthetic speech screen-access systems have a great deal in common in terms of features and functions. In fact, one trainer we spoke to points out that, in recent years, "all the software developers have started stealing from one another so that everybody's programs are beginning to look alike." Thus, it is virtually impossible to say that one product is qualitatively better than another. Just as all popular word processors provide their users with a means of blocking, moving, and deleting text, so, too, do all screen-access systems allow users to define special speech windows, for example. The way in which users perform one or another important screen-access function will vary from program to program but, if the product has gained prominence in this increasingly competitive market in the first place, chances are its developers have been careful to incorporate all critical screen-access features in either the original design or in subsequent versions of the program.

While we have previously addressed some key issues to be aware of when selecting a screen-access system (compatibility with hard- and software, conventional memory usage, customization capabilities, documentation formats), we have not yet explained the way in which a user interacts with his or her adaptive device on a day-to-day basis. That is, how, precisely, does the user gain access to the characters on the video display? What features are necessary to the user's comprehension of the data on the screen and their format? Certainly the nature of information as well as the manner in which it is interpreted differs from application to application. In a word-processing environment, information is stored in sentences, paragraphs, and pages; fields and records are the significant information storage units in database systems; and, in spreadsheet management programs, data are entered in cells, arranged in rows and columns. The blind or visually impaired computer user must be able to navigate the screen in logical accordance with its functional format, hence the need for program specific configurations. If crucial information is displayed on a status line in a word processor or if highlighted menu choices appear automatically in a spreadsheet program, the blind or visually impaired user must be made aware of this through auditory cues. Users must be able to review portions of the screen inaccessible to the system cursor (as in DOS), track lightbars, identify video attributes, and verify toggle key status quickly and easily. These functions are either performed automatically (as in the case of monitoring status lines and menu bars) when the proper configuration is loaded or by means of hot keys and/or macros. No matter what the methodology is, it is essential that the user be equipped with a means to access all important applications functions.

Vocal-eyes will automatically load the appropriate configuration or "set" file when an application is invoked provided the set files are stored in the same directory from which the speech itself was initially booted. Users who prefer to create their own set files can simply disable Vocal-eyes' "autoload" feature. While none of the other screen-access programs we examined offered an autoload feature, each did provide users with a utility to load configuration files from the command line. Thus, batch files can be written to load special configurations whenever an application is run and then reload the default configuration when exiting the program.

Although configuration files will do much of the dirty work involved in interpreting program-specific screen formats and navigation techniques, there is no simple way of customizing access to the DOS environment itself where information simply scrolls across the screen without the benefit of cursor control. Most screen-access software relies upon the ability to follow the applications cursor, enunciating characters, words, and lines as directed by the user. Since there is no cursor to follow in DOS, an alternative method of screen-access is required. Fortunately, all screen-access programs employ either a review mode, independent cursor, or both to ensure access to all portions of the screen—especially those areas to which standard cursor movement is prohibited. Whereas a sighted user would simply look at the area of interest, the blind or visually impaired user must be able to somehow designate the portion of the screen needed in order to have the information verbalized. DOS is, of course, not the only environment in which the system cursor is not controlled by the user. Many programs simply park the cursor, using alternative techniques such as reverse video to simulate cursor movement. Again, the only way to obtain full access to these applications is through the use of a secondary cursor or review mode.

Earlier we described the memory resident screen-access software as entirely "transparent" to standard applications; this means that the speech program generally sits in the background while the user interacts with the application in much the same way a sighted user does. For the most part, the adaptive device will exert little or no control over the system keyboard during normal data entry operations. Once entering review mode, however, the screen-access program is brought to the foreground and the application screen is frozen. While in review, the user may move about the screen freely—these movements will neither affect the position of the system cursor nor alter any of the data on the screen. Moreover, control of keys that are typically used by applications software is passed to the screen-access system in review. For example, the function keys, which are used quite extensively by applications such as WordPerfect, dBase, and 1-2-3, will often perform important program-specific screen-access functions in review mode. In WordPerfect, the F5 key is used to list files in the current directory. While in applications mode, the Artic user will access the WordPerfect file directory via F5 as well. Once entering review mode, however, this key will be used to invoke the Business Vision calculator. Similarly, the F1 key is used in both Lotus and dBase to obtain help, but the Vert or Vocal-eyes user who strikes this key while in review will obtain help not about the application but about the screen-access system itself. Entering review freezes the application screen, allowing the adaptive device to take temporary control of the system keyboard.

While the use of a review mode is one way to ensure noninterference with applications software, not all screen-access functions need be performed from review and, indeed, not all screen-access software includes a review feature. Neither the IBM Screen-Reader nor JAWS employs a review mode; instead, these two systems use a dual cursor design. Vocal-eyes incorporates both a review mode and independent cursor to maximize the user's screen-access capabilities. In all three cases, movement of the screen-access cursor is not limited by normal system constraints and does not affect the position of the system cursor. In this way, users may navigate the screen, "reviewing" information that is present without losing the system cursor's current position. This means that, in a word-processing environment, for example, one may reread the previous paragraph before continuing to write. Moreover, while moving the review cursor does not automatically affect the position of the system cursor, users can generally route the system cursor to the review cursor in order to modify data. If a user discovers a spelling error in a previous paragraph or wishes to add or delete information, he may route his system cursor to the proper position and make the necessary changes before continuing with his work.

Although the ability to navigate the screen fully is certainly an essential component of any speech-based adaptive software, users will also want access to a variety of voice controls and interpretation techniques. In some cases, the ability to control voice speed, pitch, and volume will be specific for the synthesizer used, but users will need to verify that such factors can be controlled at some level of operation. Similarly, users will want the ability to control the verbalization of punctuation marks, tab positions, blank spaces, lines or cells, key labels, and toggle switch status. Voice control and verbalization parameters are often set from within review mode so as to minimize key conflicts with applications software. Where no review mode is available, as with JAWS, the user will often access such features as voice speed and punctuation control through a menu system that is itself invoked by means of an unusual key combination—designed to avoid conflicts with applications software. The IBM developers took a radical approach to the question of potential key conflicts; Screen-Reader makes use of a separate eighteen-key keypad from which all screen-access functions and speech parameters are controlled. In this way, it is virtually impossible for Screen-Reader functions to interfere with the application's use of the system keyboard. However, each of the other five packages we examined, none of which employs an external keypad, managed to offer users access to a full range of speech options and navigation techniques without interfering with running applications. Keystrokes that may potentially be in conflict with applications software are generally reconfigurable so as to render the adaptive software completely unobtrusive. In the final analysis, the ability to remain virtually hidden from applications software will be the screen-access software's most critical feature.

Ease of Use

The ease with which a user acquires proficiency with one or another screen-access program will be largely due to many of the factors discussed in previous sections. Clear documentation, customization capabilities, the ability to obtain technical support, and access to an online help facility will play an important role in the learning process, but it is the intuitiveness of a program's functional features that will be of greatest concern to new users. Key assignments must make mnemonic sense in order to be retained by individuals for whom the use of a screen-access system is entirely alien. Computer-illiterate sighted users generally succeed with graphics-based systems such as the Apple Macintosh because of the memory-jogging capabilities of the icons as well as the consistency of their placement on the screen. The blind or visually impaired computer user can also benefit from spacial consistency and an intuitive keystroke design. If hot keys are grouped near one another or keystrokes used to perform similar functions are somewhat consistent, users will learn a program's idiosyncratic features quickly. Myrna Votta confirms that "people respond to something like Vocal-eyes very well because it's very intuitive . . . Control W equals word; Control L equals line."[23] The more consistency there is in a key sequence vis-à-vis its function, the easier it is to remember. If memory-jogging factors are further incorporated in the design, users will acquire speed and proficiency at an accelerated rate. Vocal-eyes' use of the sequence Ctrl (character) is not only consistent but highly intuitive given that the user need only substitute the initial character of each specific text unit in order to execute a "read current" operation: Ctrl S reads current sentence, Ctrl P reads current paragraph, and Ctrl C reads current character.

Softvert, also quite intuitive in its approach to the review mode commands, relies upon a logical layout of key sequences to perform its so-called "triplet" navigational commands. Here all keystrokes that involve horizontal movement (as with characters and words) are made with the left hand and with keys found to the left and right of the "read current" key: e.g., striking the c in review mode will read the current character, striking the x will read the previous character and striking the v will read the next character in sequence. Vertical movements (as with lines, sentences, and paragraphs) are performed with the right hand via up-and-down movements: e.g., k reads the current line, i reads the previous line, and , (comma) reads the next line of text. Unfortunately, Vert's review mode commands differ considerably from its communications mode commands so that users will need to memorize two distinct sets of key assignments in order to operate the program effectively. This disparity among communications and review mode commands is, of course, primarily due to the fact that keys such as k, i, and , are necessarily controlled by the applications software in communications mode and not by the adaptive device. Again, keys that an application regularly makes use of may be passed to the screen-access program in review without fear of conflict.

Flipper, which has a full-fledged review mode as well, also relies upon an intuitive design to help new users acquire skill with its important screen-access functions. Like many of the packages we examined, this program's advanced features may be slightly less intuitive than are the keystrokes involved in its more basic operations but, fortunately, new users need not learn these advanced functions in order to gain access to the text on the video display. Artic, although a powerfully sophisticated package, is perhaps the least intuitive of all the programs we examined. Indeed, users may find Artic's review mode operations considerably less friendly than most and may prefer to perform many screen-review functions from the normal editing screen. But if Artic's review commands initially appear somewhat less intuitive than those employed by other screen-access systems, the program compensates for this apparent shortcoming by depending primarily upon the use of standard cursor control keys (the up and down, left and right arrows) for navigational purposes. Like JAWS, Screen-Reader, and Vocal-eyes, Artic's newest release employs an independent cursor in addition to its review mode to assist users with screen-review operations in the applications mode.

As described earlier, neither JAWS nor Screen-Reader employs an actual review mode so that freezing the application in order to take temporary control of the system keyboard is somewhat tricky. In fact, Screen-Reader users need not be concerned with the system keyboard except during data entry. Remember that all voice controls, speech parameters, and screen-review functions are executed by means of the external keypad. While moving between the system keyboard and Screen-Reader keypad may cause new users a bit of difficulty at first, the pedagogical advantages to a separate keypad are significant. New users will never be confused as to whether they are executing a Screen-Reader or application command since the input device for each is distinct. Moreover, as with Softvert, Screen-Reader's keypad is logically arranged in terms of function; moving from left to right on the keypad, users will read the previous, current, and next text unit respectively. Additionally, Screen-Reader's help mode facilitates users' learning speech-specific keystrokes. As with the Kurzweil Personal Reader, this help key is available to users at all times and does not interfere with normal system operation. Indeed, users who have some familiarity with the KPR will find Screen-Reader's external keypad similar in form and function to that used by the popular reading machine. A recent Screen-Reader profile, written specifically for use with laptop computers, creates a pop-up keypad on the standard system keyboard so that users who find the external keypad clumsy and confusing may now elect not to use it at all. In any case, an essential component to Screen-Reader's ease of use is the fact that all speech functions are confined to one particular area, whether it be the external keypad or the pop-up keypad on the system keyboard.

JAWS, too, has the advantage of locational consistency. The JAWS "speech pad," as it is called, takes control of the numeric keypad of the standard desktop computer, and it is through this speech pad that JAWS users will perform common screen-review functions. Where no numeric keypad is present (as with Toshiba laptops), a special configuration file is loaded to provide users with access to screen-review functions via an alternative set of keys. The special JAWS cursor is also enabled from the numeric keypad and its movements are executed by the keys on this keypad as well. A powerful help facility and Lotus-type menu system contribute to this program's considerable ease of use.

Programs that enable the user to navigate the screen easily via keys that are intuitively named and logically arranged, and in addition facilitate the definition and reading of special speech windows, the recognition of enhanced video attributes, and that have the capabilities of interuptability and lightbar tracking will be preferable to those that lack these features. For most users, a speech program's usefulness will be closely tied to the ease with which its many features can be invoked. If key combinations are complicated and difficult to memorize, if avoiding conflicts with applications software depends upon the creation of complex configurations, if no help facility is available, and if documentation and technical support are scarce, users will rarely succeed in gaining the skill needed to function effectively in a PC environment. Before purchasing any adaptive equipment, institutions are therefore encouraged to evaluate their users' needs in tandem with the proposed equipment's capabilities. Each of the packages discussed above will perform more than adequately in most circumstances, but since each has its own strengths and weaknesses, one must be careful to weigh these strengths and weaknesses when choosing a screen-access system for use by a multiplicity of users. While the selection criteria outlined above are not exhaustive, they should prove useful in determining which speech systems will best serve your facility's needs.

Machine-Readable Formats

The widespread use of adaptive technology has contributed to the growing popularity of machine-readable or electronic texts within the print-impaired community. Texts produced in machine-readable formats are easily accessed by users of synthetic speech, screen-enlarging software, and refreshable braille systems. Moreover, producing hard copy from these so-called e-texts in braille (see chapter 3) or large print (chapter 5) is quite easy with access to the proper software packages and peripheral devices. Print-impaired computer users who rely upon auditory output systems will generally prefer machine-readable copies of informational material, reference books, and academic texts to their recorded counterparts. Given the purely sequential nature of recorded text, the ease with which e-texts are searched, referenced, and reviewed represents a vast improvement over more traditional reading techniques. In addition to the speed and ease with which machine-readable documents may be scanned, manipulated, and modified, they consume considerably less physical space in a user's library than do audiocassettes or braille books. Indeed, the introduction of CD-ROM technology in recent years has reduced the amount of storage space required for a collection of e-texts to an even greater extent. Users will find that titles such as *The Complete Works of William Shakespeare* and *The Oxford English Dictionary* as well as several encyclopedias and other reference works are readily available on CD-ROM, whereas these types of materials were rarely, if ever, made available in recorded format. Unfortunately, few public or institutional libraries and even fewer private users are equipped with the necessary hardware to access the CDs, but as the popularity of this text format increases, so too will the proliferation of the technology itself. Sony is marketing the Data Disk Man—its newest portable playback device—used to read information from CD-ROM. But for now, the availability of ASCII text files on standard 5.25- or 3.5-inch floppy disks represents a remarkable breakthrough in independent reading for most print-impaired computer users.

Because of the academic community's interest in computer assisted textual/linguistic analysis, much of the work done on the production of e-texts has been conducted in academic settings, and their use has been well underway for several years. Indeed, the original research that led to the development of Michael Hart's Project Gutenberg, whose collection now comprises over two thousand titles, started at the University of Illinois nearly twenty years ago. Projects at Dartmouth, Rutgers, Princeton, and

Georgetown have all contributed to the production of a wide variety of titles in electronic format. In fact, the Georgetown Center for Texts and Technology reports that there are currently over three hundred such projects underway in thirty countries throughout the world.[24] Thus again, as with commercially prepared spoken-word recordings, the print-impaired reader stands to benefit from a social trend by default rather than by design. The majority of the texts prepared for use by academicians will not, however, fulfill the primary reading needs of most print-impaired individuals. Fortunately, though, one of the largest organizations working to meet the reading needs of the print-impaired community, RFB (discussed earlier in this chapter in reference to audio recordings), has taken a positive stance with respect to the question of e-texts specifically designed for use by blind, visually impaired, and learning-disabled individuals.

Computerized Books for the Blind and RFB

In July of 1988, George Kerscher founded Computerized Books for the Blind (CBFB) in the basement of his Montana home with just three titles he had previously acquired from the publisher for personal use. These were Sybex's user's guides to three popular business applications: WordPerfect, dBase, and Lotus 1-2-3. Shortly thereafter, Microsoft Press gave Kerscher blanket permission to produce its publications in machine-readable format. The first employee was hired in September of that year and, as word of Kerscher's project spread through the computer-literate blind community like wildfire, so too did the organization grow. In October of 1991, CBFB and RFB merged. Kerscher is now the director of Research and Development for the new RFB.

Production and Copyright Agreements

As fully 90 percent of the e-texts generated by RFB are engineered as modifications of publishers' original source files, the production of this format starts with something of a leg up on the production of recorded books. But even though half the battle may be won by procuring publishers' source files, the documents do need to undergo a reformatting process before they are fully legible to the print-impaired reader. Often codes will appear throughout a document that indicate one or another symbol to the typesetter, but these codes would be utterly meaningless to the average reader. "If there's a symbol in a file like an 'x7234' and in the text you see an arrow pointing to the left, you have to convert that symbol to the word 'enter.' There's a logical mapping and conversion of these files."[25] The conversion process is often complicated by the fact that these typesetting conventions are not the same from one publisher to the next. Thus, the conversion program used for books published by Microsoft may not be effective with a text produced by Sybex, etc. Kerscher explains that although the codes, called "descriptive markups," tend to differ from one publishing house to another, they will generally be in standard use within each firm so that writing programs to perform the translation process on all of Microsoft's or all of Sybex's books, for example, is relatively easy.

If not particularly difficult from a technical standpoint, the conversion process can be challenging where interpretation of items such as leveled headings and meaningful changes in text size and appearance is concerned. "We're making decisions about how much information a person can actually take advantage of," Kerscher explains.[26] For example, the presence of boldfaced text might signal a particular heading to the sighted reader whereas this change in appearance might easily go unnoticed by the blind computer user who employs a speech system to access the information printed on the screen. Indeed, "bold" might not mean anything to the print-impaired individual, even if the screen-access program were designed to enunciate the word "bold" when it encountered the code. On the other hand, "heading 1" is meaningful; it does for the print-impaired individual what the bold type presumably does for the sighted reader. Thus, codes that signal significant changes in text appearance, size, or position will generally be replaced by more meaningful phrases in RFB's translation process.

Despite the conversion process, RFB's e-texts (like their recorded books) are produced with the publishers' layouts basically intact. Again, the descriptive phrases RFB substitutes for what might otherwise be cryptic codes are merely designed to provide the visually impaired user with equal access to the underlying meaning of text formats. All original pagination is retained and, wherever possible, tables, charts, and graphs are reproduced as well. In this way, not only do e-text users have access to virtually the same material as their sighted colleagues but copyright agreements are not broached since the text has not been essentially modified. Given the relative youth of the electronic text format, virtually no case law has yet been established to address issues of copyright infringement adequately. One view is that "current notions of copyright will have to be heavily modified to be of use in an electronic environment. Proponents of this position feel that electronic text is too easily mutable, too subject to unauthorized change and redistribution to be governed by the same laws that apply to print publications."[27] Although there are laws that expressly prohibit the reproduction of e-texts purchased from RFB, users are bound by little more than their honor. No special equipment is needed to access the texts and the disks are not copy-protected. Thus, the ease with which Kerscher has managed to obtain publishers' source files may be indicative of an increased awareness of the need for accessible text formats. He is, however, quick to point out that legislation passed in 1988 requires hard- and software manufacturers to provide blind and visually-impaired users with accessible copies of their product documentation. It is perhaps not surprising, then, that most of RFB's current e-text library is composed of computer-related texts.

The RFB Collection and Text Distribution

In fact, the reasons for RFB's current e-text holdings being primarily concentrated in the area of computer technology are manifold. Although the 508 bill, which mandated equal access to computer product documentation, certainly contributed to Kerscher's ability to obtain publishers' source files, the production of this type of material in electronic format was originally an outgrowth of Kerscher's own needs. Since he was a graduate student in computer science when he founded CBFB, many of the texts he sought to procure were related to that discipline. Moreover, he explains that the individuals who expressed interest in the service during its early days were predominately computerphiles. Finally, unlike many publishing houses, most computer companies tend to produce their publications themselves; they do not generally use outside compositors so that there is an increased availability of source files. But as RFB's membership is diverse, there can be no doubt that the organization will expand its collection in untold directions during the coming years. Kerscher describes research into the logical translation of scientific and mathematical notation. And already there are plans to begin producing scholarly periodicals and academic journals, keeping in line with RFB's longtime commitment to the educational needs of the print-impaired student and professional.

All RFB members were automatically registered for CBFB services and vice versa following the 1991 merger. Anyone who registers with RFB today gains immediate access to both the collection of audiocassettes and of e-texts. To obtain information about either of the services, contact RFB's customer service department at the toll-free number provided in appendix A. Interested users who have not yet acquired information about the collection of e-texts should request the e-kit that is distributed free of charge to registered members. It should be noted that, unlike the audio recordings, RFB's e-texts are not borrowed but purchased. Pricing information as well as payment procedures are explained in detail in the e-kit.

Current Trends and Future Developments

At present, the format of RFB's e-texts is not particularly glamorous. Each chapter of a given book is stored in an ordinary ASCII text file as is the table of contents and index. Users may use READ.COM (described earlier), or the DOS TYPE command to scan the material in each file from the command line or, alternatively, they may import the files into their favorite word processor. But, like many of the individuals involved in the production and dissemination of machine-readable texts, Kerscher believes that the next important step in providing users with full access to RFB's e-texts lies in the development of software that would facilitate the scanning process. "We need software that is going to have sophisticated searching capabilities, give us the ability to move easily from the table of contents into the book, easily from the index back into the book, allow us to retrace our steps so that when it says 'see page 192' we can hop to page 192 and then back to where we were. We need to be able to leave bookmarks and we need software that would allow us to organize not only one book but an entire library," he explains. [28]

Indeed, the development of software packages designed for use with electronic texts is well underway in the private sector. Bellcore has developed a program called Superbook, IBM has a package called Bookman, and The Electronic Text Corporation distributes something called Wordcruncher. Each of these applications has been specifically designed to help the user search through electronic texts quickly and easily and to, in effect, offer their users all the advantages of a printed text in a paperless environment. As Reva Basch points out, "the very existence of software like this, not to mention the involvement of major players like Ma Bell and Big Blue, is an indication that electronic texts are being taken seriously at least for some applications." [29] It is important to recognize, however, that the software packages developed by these major corporations are designed with a sighted user in mind. Chances are, they will not serve the needs of the print-impaired computer user fully. In fact, it seems likely that the user interface may be problematic for speech-based screen-access systems. Kerscher's software will, on the other hand, be engineered with the needs of the blind user as its first priority. Moreover, he anticipates cooperation from the various screen-access software companies in devising program-specific configuration files to work with RFB's new e-text software.

Recall that publishers' source files used in the production of RFB's e-texts undergo a conversion process in which all meaningful symbols and font changes are translated to descriptive text; similarly, all layout and design features aimed at pleasing the readers' visual aesthetic sense are stripped before the book is ready for distribution. Again, changes in size and appearance, placement of text, and lines of asterisks or other symbols may contribute to the readability of a document for the sighted reader, but such visual apparatuses are, at best, lost on the print-impaired user and, at worst, may interfere with his comprehension of the text. Thus, commercial firms involved in the production of electronic texts may inadvertently diminish the texts' primary usefulness to the blind or visually impaired reader when they attempt to spruce up their formats with visually stimulating devices. For the time being, texts stored in ordinary ASCII format may be best suited to use by blind and visually-impaired users since ASCII code represents no potential conflict with standard speech configurations. The Reader Project, an effort to distribute machine-readable texts in compressed form to blind and visually impaired computer users via modem, did not achieve the level of success its creators might have hoped because, in large part, of the fact that readers were compelled to use the project's proprietary scanning software in order to access the documents. While this software offered users advanced search capabilities, the ability to leave electronic bookmarks, and a facility for setting up special reading windows, it was not fully compatible with all adaptive software and severely limited users' independent choice. Kerscher asserts that RFBers will always have the option of accessing his e-texts as normal ASCII files even after the development and distribution of the special scanning software.

The Graphical User Interface and Speech

Up until now, our discussion of synthetic speech screen-access has focused exclusively on IBM and compatible systems—specifically, on MS-DOS based machines. MS-DOS is a character-based operating system. Information that is to be put on the computer screen is stored in a portion of the computer's memory called the "display text buffer." As the information in the display text buffer is stored in ASCII code, the adaptive TSR can simply look to the buffer for the data to be verbalized. Computers such as the Apple Macintosh use an entirely different screen-rendering architecture. Information that is to be displayed on the computer screen is bit-mapped to the computer's memory and then literally painted on the screen. This means that rather than storing the ASCII value for the letter a, for example, in a text buffer, a graphics-based computer will print a series of dots (called pixels) to the computer's memory, the precise position and formation of which will then be replicated on the video display itself. These pixels, when grouped together, will represent an a to the sighted user but, to the screen-access system which relies upon an ASCII value to translate the character in question, the pixels are meaningless, completely uninterpretable. This pixel by pixel screen-writing method allows for a graphical user interface (GUI) in that iconigraphic images, special fonts, and proportional lettering may be easily displayed on the screen but, of course, there is no way for standard speech-based screen-access systems to decipher these images. Users of GUI-based systems will immediately recognize a second, equally formidable barrier to access for blind and visually impaired users vis-à-vis the use of a mouse as an input device. In a DOS environment, commands are entered from the system keyboard as text strings; with GUIs, users move a mouse to the desired icon and simply click the button to execute various commands. For sighted computer users, the mouse used in conjunction with memory-jogging icons adds up to an extremely friendly operating system, but for the blind user the GUIs can represent a veritable minefield of confusion and potential disaster.

Given the choice, most synthetic speech users would probably prefer to avoid the GUIs altogether, but doing so is becoming increasingly difficult. Not only has the Apple Macintosh become as popular as the IBM PC in most professional and academic settings, but MicroSoft's introduction of Windows several years ago and IBM's having jumped on the GUI bandwagon as well with OS/2 and Presentation Manager (PM) would indicate that character-based machines are truly a dying breed. Fortunately, steps are being taken to ensure that the blind and visually impaired computer user will not be locked out of the GUI revolution as was originally feared.

Berkeley Systems, Inc. (BSI), developed OutSpoken in 1989 to provide speech users with access to the Mac. OutSpoken uses the Mac's built-in synthesizer to produce the sounds of English and relies on a so-called "interception" technique to virtually circumvent the GUI altogether. Regarding the mouse, OutSpoken users will simulate mouse navigation using the numeric keypad on the system keyboard. When an icon is encountered, the word "icon" is voiced and then a verbal description is given: e.g., "trash can." While the system does not yet provide users with true access to all the benefits of the GUI environment, OutSpoken's developers are presently working in tandem with Dr. Gregg Vanderheiden, director of Wisconsin's Trace Research and Development Center, to incorporate a multisensory approach to screen navigation using tactile, three-dimensional sound cues. As Vanderheiden and his colleagues point out, "specifically the problem with using speech-based solutions only is that it is difficult to keep track continuously of where things are on the screen."[30]

Engineers and software developers at IBM's Thomas J. Watson Research Institute in New York have been working on a new version of Screen-Reader that will run with OS/2-PM and, in a recent Screen-Reader newsletter, encouraging announcements were made regarding the project's progress. The company has been beta-testing the software with its employees and other Screen-Reader-OS/2 users with considerable success, but although the prototype is currently being demonstrated at adaptive technology conferences and trade shows, the product is not yet commercially available. Like OutSpoken, Screen-Reader/PM uses an interception technique. Richard Schwerdtfeger, one of the IBM researchers, explains that text, which is bit-mapped onto the computer's memory, is modified for synthetic speech output via the maneuverings of an off-screen model (OSM). The OSM will create the illusion of a conventional display text buffer so that the speech program is able to interpret information stored there.[31] But again, the use of an OSM to enable speech-based access to any graphics-oriented environment should, according to Boyd, Boyd, and Vanderheiden, be regarded as little more than a temporary accommodation.

Advantages

The interception techniques described above fall short of providing full access to the GUIs since these techniques do not enable blind and visually impaired users to take advantage of the very qualities that define the Mac's user-friendliness. In their argument in favor of a multisensory solution, Boyd, Boyd, and Vanderheiden assert that "the single sensory strategy does not provide the full benefits of the scanning, browsing, and memory-jogging functions of the graphical user interface or the full benefits of locational and formatting information."[32] If the GUIs are truly here to stay, then, as Jay Leventhal concedes, "we've got to deal with them."[33] "Dealing with them" involves the development of screen-access systems that do not simply circumvent the GUI but offer blind and visually impaired users a user-friendly alternative to MS-DOS based machines. The GUI environment should do for the blind or visually impaired individual what it does for a sighted user: facilitate all levels of computer operation as well as augment participation in activities such as desktop publishing, musical composition, and graphics design.

One might naturally assume that the graphical user interface would be of greatest use to the learning-disabled. Indeed, the advantages of a graphics-based system for those who have difficulty with text (command) processing are obvious, but important spacial concepts relative to mouse navigation techniques may occasionally prove problematic with this group of users. Moreover, some learning-disabled individuals will have conceptual difficulty with iconic representations of objects and tasks. In these cases, the interception techniques of today's speech-based access systems may be highly effective.

In general, print-impaired individuals who respond well to metaphor will have little trouble mastering the principals involved in the graphical user interface. Moreover, the consistency with which all Macintosh applications are constructed contributes to the ease with which blind users can memorize screen-layout. Navigating an applications screen with or without a mouse is greatly simplified by the locational consistency of functionally similar entities. Again, current speech-based screen-access systems may not be fully adequate where the GUIs are concerned, but ongoing research at places like BSI, Trace, and IBM will ensure the continued participation of blind, visually impaired, and learning-disabled individuals in the technological revolution.

Notes

1. *That All May Read: Library Service for the Blind and Physically Handicapped* (Washington, D.C.: Library of Congress, National Library Service for the Blind and Physically Handicapped, 1983), 80.
2. Ibid., 79.
3. Ibid., 87.
4. See appendix A for a list of publishers and distributors through whom these materials might be obtained.
5. See chapter 3 for additional details on Pratt-Smoot and the historical development of the NLS. Also, the library service's development is chronicled in *That All May Read: Library Service for the Blind and Physically Handicapped* (Washington, D.C.: Library of Congress, National Library Service for the Blind and Physically Handicapped, 1983).
6. Again, the reader is referred to appendix A for a comprehensive list of these independent distributors.
7. Note that major bibliographic utilities, such as RLIN and OCLC, are also potential sources for identifying spoken word recordings.
8. Susan Mosakowski, director of the talking book recording studio, New York Regional Library for the Blind, personal interview with Dawn M. Suvino, New York, January 27, 1992.
9. Ibid.
10. Laurie Facciarossa, RFB public information officer, telephone interview with Dawn M. Suvino, January 27, 1992.
11. Eunice Lovejoy, "History and Standards" in *That All May Read*, 3.
12. It should be noted that the NLS does produce a number of magazines in audio format. However, these are monthly periodicals and, in fact, often subscribers do not receive the texts in a timely fashion. Rather, the July issue of one or another popular magazine may not reach the subscriber's mailbox before September or October.
13. Franklin S. Cooper, "Research on Reading Machines for the Blind" in *Blindness: Modern Approaches to the Unseen Environment*, edited by Paul A. Zahl (Princeton, N.J.: Princeton Univ. Pr., 1950), 512.
14. Cooper's description of the early events leading to the development of the first electronic reading machines is fascinating. Readers wishing to learn more about these events and subsequent research at Haskins and RCA should consult Cooper's text. His bibliography includes a number of seminal articles on the subject as well.
15. Louise Melton, "Mister Impossible: Ray Kurzweil," *Computers & Electronics* 22 (July 1984): 40-49.
16. The reader is referred to two articles published in the *Journal of Academic Librarianship:* Diane W. Kazlauskas, Sharon T. Weaver, and William R. Jones, "Kurzweil Reading Machine: a Study of Usage Patterns," (January 1987): 356–58; Gerald Jahoda and Elizabeth A. Johnson, "The Use of the Kurzweil Reading Machine in Academic Libraries" (May 1987): 99–101.
17. The reader is referred to chapter 2 for a more detailed discussion of optical

character recognition technology and to appendix B for specific product information.

18. Myrna Votta, New York Association for the Blind, personal interview with Dawn M. Suvino, New York, March 6, 1992.
19. See appendix B for a more complete resource listing.
20. Note that the DOS 5 ANSI.SYS may cause conflicts with many speech-based screen-access software systems. Users who wish to upgrade to the new version of the operating system are advised to use an earlier version of the device driver. As problems have been reported with the DOS 4 ANSI.SYS as well, we would suggest using the DOS 3.3 ANSI.SYS.
21. Myrna Votta, personal interview, New York, March 6, 1992.
22. J. Leventhal, AFB National Technology Center, personal interview with Dawn M. Suvino, New York, January 22, 1992.
23. Myrna Votta, personal interview, New York, March 6, 1992.
24. Reva Basch, "Books On-line: Visions, Plans, and Perspectives for Electronic Texts," *Online* 15 (July 1991): 14.
25. George Kerscher, telephone interview with Dawn M. Suvino, New York, February 13, 1992.
26. Ibid.
27. Reva Basch, "Books Online," 17.
28. George Kerscher, telephone interview, February 13, 1992.
29. Reva Basch, "Books Online," 20.
30. Lawrence H. Boyd, Wesley L. Boyd, and Gregg. C. Vanderheiden, "The Graphical User Interface: Crisis, Danger and Opportunity," *Journal of Visual Impairment and Blindness* 84 (Dec. 1990): 501.
31. Richard S. Schwerdtfeger, "Making the GUI Talk," *Byte* (Dec. 1991): 118.
32. Boyd, Boyd, and Vanderheiden, "The Graphical User Interface."
33. J. Leventhal, personal interview, New York, January 22, 1992.

Chapter Five

Materials and Technology for Low-Vision Readers

Thus far our attention has been focused on materials and technologies developed for and used primarily by readers who are blind or whose visual impairment is quite severe. Only the blind use the tactile reading methods described in chapter 3. In the case of the audio-based text sources (cassettes and synthetic speech) profiled in chapter 4, we have seen that people with learning disabilities also use and benefit from some of the same technology used by people with visual impairments; by listening to a text as they read the printed version, many learning-disabled readers can increase not only their reading speed but also their comprehension and retention of textual content.

The blind will probably constitute just a small fraction of the total population served by most libraries, with the obvious exception of those facilities designed specifically for this segment of the population. Most librarians will encounter many more readers with some degree of vision, whose "visual acuity," however, disallows independent access to regular size print. Of the estimated fourteen million Americans with visual impairments, the vast majority are somewhere within the latter group.

One might expect that, compared with braille and audio publications, large print materials would provide the earliest examples of print adaptation for readers with vision disabilities. Braille texts required the development of an entirely new system for the transcription of written language. The development of audio texts required advanced technology with an even more recent history. Surprisingly, however, of these three formats the widespread use of large print books by people with limited vision has the shortest history.

The earliest printed texts were produced in type that would not have been legible to a considerable portion of the adult population without the aid of the earliest adaptive technology—eye glasses. Some historians of the book propose that if corrective lenses had not been invented *before* the advent of modern printing, typography might have taken an entirely different course. Without corrective lenses, which guaranteed an adult audience able to read what we now call "conventional type size," the earliest books might have been produced in larger type. In an essay titled "Spectacles 100 Years Before and 100 Years After the Invention of Printing," professor Otto Hallauer, a Swiss doctor and historian of medicine, noted that "the spread of printing throughout many countries encouraged the desire and need to read; after this invention a greater demand for spectacles must have arisen among older people."[1] Indeed, many individuals are able to comfortably read the print of this book only with the aid of corrective lenses.

Like braille and other embossed texts, large type books were originally designed for use in schools by visually impaired readers. Students in the special "sight-saving classes" for the visually impaired in the public schools of Cleveland were provided the first texts in this format by Dr. Robert Irwin in 1913.[2] It was not until the 1960s, however, that the commercial publishing industry entered the field of large print book and magazine production. The period from 1964, when the first seven large print books were produced commercially in England, to 1972, when industry growth began to level off, have in fact been described as the years of the "Large Print Revolution."[3]

Following our discussion of the large print publishing industry and its relationship to libraries and low-vision readers, we will explore the in-house production of large print materials. Each of the electronic information sources discussed throughout this monograph can be adapted to the needs of individuals with low vision. Laser printers allow the production of paper copy of machine-readable information sources in the print size preferred by individual readers. For the reader who does not want or need a paper copy of a text, large print computer displays provide independent access to the contents of the computer screen, magnifying characters up to sixteen times the computer monitor's normal print size.

Large type reading materials will be just one of several innovations considered in this chapter. A number of other developments, such as the use of closed-circuit television (CCTV) technology for the enlargement of printed materials, have had a tremendous impact on the ability of low-vision readers to access standard size printed materials without assistance from librarians or readers. Many libraries already provide access to such enlargement devices for their print-impaired population. And unlike much of the "big-ticket" adaptive equipment discussed throughout this monograph, CCTV enlargement devices are inexpensive enough to be considered for purchase by individuals as well as libraries operating with very limited budgets.

In relation to CCTV technology, other low-tech aids and services will also be identified and described. Most libraries already have technology in place that can benefit a large number of low-vision readers. Most microform readers (and copiers), for example, allow numerous enlargement options, including print much larger than that used in conventional large print materials (usually limited to 16 or 18 points in size). The illuminated, enlarged image of microform newspapers, magazines, and books is actually the preferred format of a significant number of low-vision readers who are comfortable with the technology required to access microform publications.

Surprisingly little research has been conducted into the potential use of microfilm and fiche by visually impaired readers. In one relatively early study of microfiche and CCTV use by low-vision readers, however, it was demonstrated that many individuals with low vision in fact achieve faster reading speeds with microfiche rather than with other optical aids (such as CCTV devices).[4]

Torsten Andersson, the Swedish researcher who conducted this study for the Uppsala School of Education, urges the rehabilitation community to promote the use of microfiche as a low-vision reading aid.

The appearance and rapid proliferation of personal computers in the 1980s did not leave low-vision readers unaffected. Computer-based screen enlargement technology has extended the independence of low-vision readers vis-à-vis regular-sized print reading materials. Introduced in the early 1980s, these adaptive software and hardware products allow the visually impaired reader to access portions of the computer display in large print. Some systems offer "split-screen" access to both hard copy (using the CCTV technology mentioned above) and computer text.

We will conclude this chapter with a discussion of the reference librarian's responsibility to the low-vision patron. Before going on to discuss any of the adaptive devices and accessible formats we have mentioned, we will describe our target population, focusing on definitions of terms such as "visual acuity," "low vision," and "legal blindness."

The Reader with Limited Vision

As early as 1916 Robert Irwin, pioneer in the field of education and rehabilitation of the blind, began questioning some of the methods and materials used to educate school-age children with visual impairments. In a proposal and rationale for "sight-saving classes," geared toward low-vision students in the public schools, he notes that many such students enter schools for the blind where they are "usually instructed as totally blind children. After long and persistent effort on the part of both teacher and pupil, some facility in finger reading (of braille) is acquired. This method of reading seldom becomes easy to this class of pupils, and when left to themselves they soon succumb to the temptation to read the braille with their eyes."[5] Some low-vision students undoubtedly derived some benefit from learning braille, particularly those who would eventually lose their sight completely. Today, by comparison, the vast majority of readers with low vision are encouraged to use whatever vision they have. This change in the attitude of vision rehabilitation professionals toward residual vision, coupled with advances in corrective lenses and low-vision adaptive technology aids, has contributed immeasurably to the independence of this chapter's target population.

The criteria used by the National Library Service to determine eligibility for service and materials have been detailed in chapter 3: *Visually impaired* individuals are considered eligible for NLS service if their "visual acuity . . . is 20/200 or less in the better eye with correcting lenses, or whose widest diameter of visual field subtends an angular distance no greater than 20 degrees." While something of an oversimplification, individuals with visual acuity of 20/200 are able to see at a distance of 20 feet what those with normal sight can see at approximately 200 feet. Those whose "visual field subtends an angular distance of no greater than 20 degrees," are severely limited in their field of vision, and may have a condition referred to as "tunnel vision." In 1988, the American Foundation for the Blind reported that approximately 600,000 Americans are registered as legally blind. The same source indicates that "professionals in the field estimate that the number of legally blind persons is really three times the number who are registered as such."[6]

The NLS criteria defining visual impairment also define "legal blindness" in the United States. Interestingly, visual acuity conditions governing legally blind status and eligibility for associated benefits differ widely on an international level. In one study of the global incidence of blindness, the World Health Organization identified sixty-five different definitions of "legal blindness" which encompassed many different allowable levels of acuity.[7]

The past few decades have seen a revolutionary change in rehabilitation professionals' views of vision and visual impairment in general. Much of the research conducted by Natalie Barraga and others in the use of residual vision has prompted the rehabilitation community to begin viewing low vision as a "functional state rather than a medical diagnosis."[8] "Historically, the tendency has been to rely upon acuity measurements for distinction between those eligible for service and those for whom no legal or medical justification can be made for need of services."[9] Given our penchant as a society for the empirical, it is not surprising that measurement of visual acuity should have such a stronghold on our concept of visual impairment. Acuity is, after all, fairly easily and reliably quantifiable. In a 1975 study on the use of residual vision by adults with severe visual impairments, Dr. Barraga urged educators and other rehabilitation professionals to stop "focusing upon a medical measurement or a legal eligibility factor, and to begin giving attention to the question: What does this person need to learn, or to what does he need to adapt in relation to his own life?"[10] This trend toward utilization of residual vision has done much to encourage the development of and secure an audience for accessible-format reading materials, as well as low- and high-tech adaptive reading devices for the low-vision reader.

Dr. Robert Irwin's use of large type in his public school sight-saving classes must be viewed as an isolated occurrence rather than the beginning of a national trend; large print books did not gain widespread acceptance until the 1940s, when the American Printing House for the Blind and other publishers began mass production of educational texts in this accessible format. We will next look at the criteria that have been established for large print book publishing and review the history of the large print publishing industry before beginning our discussion of the library's role vis-à-vis the low-vision reader.

Large Print

Print size is measured in "points," from the top of the tallest letter to the bottom of the lowest: for example, from the top of the capital T to the "tail" of the lowercase y. Each "point," or unit of type, measures 1/72 inch. Type that measures one inch high is, therefore, 72-point type. Most regular-sized print publications are set in 10- or 12-point type, which is less than 1/6 inch in height. For a visual comparison of various type sizes, see figure 6.

While most regular-sized printed publications are produced in 10- to 12-point type, there are some that utilize type only 8 points in size, or smaller. Some important reference sources fall within the latter category. The *Arts and Humanities*, *Social Science*, and *Science Citation* indexes, for example, are printed in 5-point type. Some readers who can comfortably read regular size type might need a magnifying glass in order to effectively use materials printed in such small type; at the very least, the accessible library will make magnifying glasses available in the reference room and for use throughout the library.

Today, large print materials are most commonly produced in 16- or 18-point type. For the purposes of the National Library Service's postage-free distribution of materials, type 14 points or larger is considered "large print." In addition to print size, some other attributes that affect the readability of large print materials include strong contrast between paper and ink, simplicity of typeface, and increased line "leading" (pronounced "ledding"), or spacing between the lines of text. Dark ink on white, nonglare paper is considered most effective for reading materials in large type.

The American Printing House for the Blind, mentioned earlier in connection with braille textbook publishing, began producing large print educational materials in 1946. Stanwix House, another major publisher of accessible format texts, soon followed the lead of APH, and began producing large print materials primarily for elementary schoolchildren.[11] Production of large print educational materials gained momentum in the 1950s

This is 10-point type.

This is 12-point type.

This is 14-point type.

This is 18-point type.

This is 24-point type.

This is 36-point type.

This is 48-point type.

Figure 6. Examples of print sizes, measured in "points." Most large print books and magazines are printed in 14-, 16-, or 18-point type.

when Lorraine Marchi began a volunteer collaborative effort to produce materials for students with low vision. Marchi's nonprofit organization, National Aid for Visually Handicapped (NAVH), continues to address the needs of the low-vision population, and is the only association devoted exclusively to their needs.

It wasn't until 1965, however, that observers of the publishing industry identified the enormous potential *adult* audience for large print reading materials. Joel A. Roth, addressing the concerns of low-vision readers, referred to the adult low-vision population as a "four-million reader market which sits patiently in the half-light of limited vision, waiting for the publishing industry to meet its needs. Considerable energy has been focused on the needs of the child with limited vision, but low-vision readers under 20 years of age account for only one-eighth of the four million Americans with low vision."[12]

While APH and other government subsidized producers of accessible textbooks had been producing large print materials since the 1940s, it was not until 1964 that commercial publishers began addressing the needs of the rapidly increasing audience for large print. First introduced in 1964 by Ulverscroft, a British publisher, large type materials had become less expensive to produce as a result of innovations in the printing industry—notably, the use of photo-offset enlargement and printing techniques. Publications in the Ulverscroft series were photographically enlarged to twice the size of the original imprint. "In 1971, G. K. Hall became the first American large print publisher to produce books by the photocomposition method—a faster means of reprinting current bestsellers and other contemporary titles. More importantly, photocomposition eliminated the distortions and imperfections of the photo-offset process."[13] Remember that the earliest large type books and magazines had to be typeset, resulting in very high production costs. Photomechanical reproduction should thus be seen as the technology that rendered production of large print materials commercially viable for publishing companies, which are in the business, after all, of making money.

Microfilm and fiche, a relatively young technology in the 1960s, also had an impact on large print book production. A number of micropublishers began offering large print hard copy output of microform books and magazines "on demand." While the titles produced were more expensive than commercial, mass-produced large print publications, the early micropublishing industry extended the options available to the reader (or library) in search of materials in large type.

Once commercial production of a variety of materials in large print finally got under way, the audience for large print materials was quickly shifted from school-aged children with visual impairments to aging readers, and this trend has grown steadily over the past three decades. Several reasons have been offered for the continuing growth in the market for large print books and magazines. Medical advances, in terms of preventive care as well as our ability to cure previously fatal diseases, have had the effect of prolonging the average lifespan of the general population; this aging of the population has produced increasing numbers of elderly people in need of specialized library and other services. One of the primary and natural consequences of the aging process is, of course, the loss of visual acuity. It has been suggested that the primary audience for large print will continue to be the elderly, many of whom, being on fixed incomes, will look to libraries for reading materials in this relatively expensive format.[14]

The National Library Service does not produce materials in large print for a number of reasons. In our examination of recorded texts, we saw that the NLS role in the production of accessible text formats has been made possible as a result of special copyright agreements with publishers. The special playback equipment required for NLS audio texts assures publishers that only NLS patrons will use the cassette or flexible disk, affecting profits from the regular printed version of the text minimally. The rights to produce a braille version of a book are freely given, on the assumption that only blind people will know braille, and sales of the print version of the title will not be significantly affected. Large type books and magazines present an entirely different situation; accessible to readers of the regular edition of any, large print surely poses a threat to sales of those texts. As mentioned earlier, materials acquired by libraries may, however, be sent postage free if they are printed in type that is 14 points or larger. Most public libraries acquire books in large print, and these may be shipped to homebound patrons at no cost to the library. The New York Public Library, for example, has a "Books by Mail Program" through which home-bound patrons can receive materials by mail. While all "Books by Mail" are shipped at no cost to the patron, only the large print titles qualify for "Free Matter for the Blind" postage status. Mailing costs for regular size print materials become part of the regular operating costs of the program, i.e., payable by New York Public Library funds.[15]

The large print publishing industry expects growth to increase throughout the '90s, and the mainstream publishing community is beginning to exploit the potential for profit in a number of ways. In the past, most publishers simply licensed the large print production rights of individual titles to large print specialty publishers, like G. K. Hall. Some major trade publishers are beginning to enter the field of large print production on their own, offering large print editions of new works simultaneously with the regular edition, usually at a slightly higher price. Large publishing houses, like Random House and Doubleday, have fledgling large print divisions that cater to an adult low-vision audience. Similarly, bookstore chains and even the Book-of-the-Month club offer large print selections to the rapidly growing number of large print readers.[16]

Libraries and Low-Vision Readers

Librarians' interest in the reading needs of people with low vision dates from 1923, when the American Library Association began publication of *Books for Tired Eyes: A List of Books in Large Print.* Compiled by Charlotte

Matson of the Minneapolis Public Library, *Books for Tired Eyes* was updated several times until the 1950s, and was supplemented by several public library systems' inventories of their large print holdings.[17]

In the 1960s, just two years after the first commercial large print titles were produced in England, a major study of the potential *adult* audience for large print books and magazines, made possible by a Library Services and Construction Act grant, was undertaken by the New York Public Library. With just forty-one titles in its collection, the Large Print Book Project set out to study the use of large print publications by the library's adult readership over the course of a two-year period. Until the 1960s, when commercial publishers began producing large print books, materials were created almost exclusively for children. The Large Print Book Project concluded that there is a significantly large potential adult audience for large type books and magazines, but noted that reaching this audience can be difficult for a variety of reasons. "Many have stopped reading and have stopped using the library; many live in institutions and are therefore cut off from public services and, in general, many lack mobility owing to sight limitation, age, or a complexity of health problems."[18]

The problem of developing and maintaining "well-balanced" large print collections was also addressed by the NYPL Large Print Project. Remember that the industry was in its infancy, and that only a fraction of the regular size print titles on the market were also available in large print. In order to satisfy the needs and interests of its adult clientele, the New York Public Library added many titles to its large print collection (at considerable cost) by the photographic reproduction and enlargement service of microformat publishers mentioned earlier. The project report indicates that titles selected for enlargement "proved to be the most popular during the Project's duration,"[19] undoubtedly because selectors had a keen awareness of their patrons' reading habits and tastes.

Large Print Reference Sources

Several reference sources are available to assist librarians in the selection and acquisition of large print books and magazines. The major large type "books in print," Bowker's annual *Complete Directory of Large Print Books and Serials*, provides access to over 5,500 book entries produced by close to sixty publishers (in its 1990 edition). In order to qualify for inclusion in the *Complete Directory*, books and magazines must be set in type 14 points or larger, and point size is indicated for each entry. Access is provided by subject, textbook subject, and children's subject indexes. Title and author indexes allow the user to identify specific items to determine whether or not a large print version of a desired item exists, and, if so, how one may acquire a copy.

The American Printing House for the Blind offers a number of large print textbooks for students at all levels. APH's *Central Catalog* lists the large print holdings of this publisher of educational materials, along with braille and audio tape texts. The online version of the APH Catalog, APH-CARL, is also available to librarians serving low-vision patrons. For a more comprehensive description of APH-CARL, see chapter 3.

While the National Library Service does not produce materials in large print, most of its own informational publications and brochures are made available in this format. The NLS reference circular, *Reading Materials in Large Type*, available free of charge, provides a good introduction to large type materials, and identifies major publishers and reference works available in type 14 points or larger. Last updated in 1987, this guide also identifies large print magazines and devotional materials available from a number of commercial as well as not-for-profit publishers.

Unlike braille and recorded texts, which are for the most part excluded from the National Union Catalog as well as the major bibliographic utilities, large print reading materials can be identified using both OCLC and RLIN. Library of Congress cataloging rules stipulate that large type books be identified as such. A subject search of the RLIN database yields over 27,000 records for books in large print.[20] Interestingly, serial records contain no such indication of format. The *New York Times Large Type Weekly*, for example, can be located only if the exact title is known, or if the RLIN Serials file is searched by keywords "large" and (print or type). Incidentally, there are very few major periodicals produced in large print. Bruce Massis, librarian at the Jewish Guild for the Blind, points out that large type editions of the *New York Times* (weekly) and the *Reader's Digest* are the exception.[21]

A number of large print reference sources are available for purchase by libraries interested in extending access to readers with low vision. See appendix A for a directory of the major large print publishers; a list of selected reference sources available in large type can be found in appendix C.

Production of Materials in Large Print

Prior to the introduction of the photocopy machine in the 1960s, libraries simply collected materials and made them available for use in the library, or on short-term loan. The concept of making a reproduction of printed material was really quite revolutionary and has had a tremendous impact on the way people use libraries and conduct research; for better or worse, most libraries have become production facilities of a sort. With the advent of computer technology in the 1980s, many libraries extended their role in the area of materials production by providing access to microcomputers for a variety of functions, from database searching to word processing. "Where's the photocopy machine?" and "Can I get a printout?" are increasingly common requests at reference desks in most libraries.

Many modern photocopy machines offer enlargement and reduction options, and most such machines are capable of handling paper of varying sizes. Photocopy machines may be used to enlarge type to just about any size, but the size of the page must increase accordingly. Also, depending upon the quality of the material to be copied, as well as the machine itself, type that is radically enlarged on a photocopy machine will lose some degree of clarity (see figure 7). Certainly, for the library serving a large number of readers with low vision, promotional materials produced in large print on a photocopy machine will prove adequate. In addition to supplying vital information such as schedule and programming information in a form that will be appreciated by people with limited vision, the library will also be promoting its own interest in serving the needs of its print-impaired population.

Computer-based text holds even greater potential for high-quality large print output. For the library equipped with a laser printer, most electronic texts can be easily produced in the reader's preferred type size. For production of large print materials, the laser printer has several advantages over the photocopy machine. First, type size can be changed and the text reformatted so that regular size paper may be used. The downloaded text of an article from an online database, for example, can be produced in just minutes, with good, clear print on 8 1/2-by-11-inch paper. Many word processing programs also allow subtle variations in some printing attributes that are considered important in the production of large print. WordPerfect, for example, allows modifications in line "leading," or spacing between lines of text. Since the earliest appearance of large print publications, most research indicates that increased line leading contributes to the readability of these materials. For an example of the effect of increased leading of an 18-point text, see figures 8 and 9. Often, new users look for promotional information and subject-specific pathfinders to guide them in their use of the library and its collections. Large type versions of library information bulletins are easily produced on a computer with a minimal amount of reformatting, and serve to alert readers to the library's commitment to its disabled clientele.

In our discussion of braille production in chapter 3, we saw that regular printed materials can easily be converted to machine-readable files. Using the Optical Character Recognition equipment described in chapter 2, readers can use the power of the personal computer and the clarity of laser printing technology to produce very high quality documents in the point size of their choice. Remember that when we scan printed sources, the resulting ASCII text file can be edited with a word processor for output in any number of adaptive formats, including large print. Figure 10 illustrates the steps involved in the conversion of an encyclopedia article in 10-point type into an 18-point document. Note that, depending largely on the quality of the source document, scanned materials are rarely flawless, and may require some editing before an acceptable large print version can be produced.

WASHINGTON

FOR 80 of his 85 years, Kenneth M. Russell has nurtured a special love for natural pearls. As a child he helped his father rummage for them in shellfish from the Mississippi, and his parents made the down payment on a house with money from a $600 pearl.

As an adult, he has collected thousands of pearls, a few each year, and devoted much of his spare time to studying their mysterious luster. Mr. Russell, now a retired trade association executive who lives in Bethesda, Md., says the Bible refers to pearls 10 times, while diamonds rate only 3 mentions. "A diamond is like a piece of glass," he said. "Pearls are soft and have a quiet elegance. It is the one gem that cannot be improved by man."

Mr. Russell has patented a device that he says makes it much easier to distinguish natural pearls from cultured pearls, which are grown by placing tiny granules of clamshell

Figure 7. Newsprint enlarged on a photocopy machine. Note the lack of clarity compared to laser copy large print (see figures 8 and 9).

This is an example of 18 point text, with regular "line leading." Line leading (pronounced "ledding") is the space between lines of text. The term refers to the line of lead that was used by typesetters when preparing a page for printing.

Figure 8. 18-point text, regular line leading

This is also 18 point type, but with an

increase in line leading. The added space

between lines can make text much clearer

for readers with low vision. Most popular

word processing programs allow for modi-

fications in line leading.

Figure 9. 18-point text, increased line leading

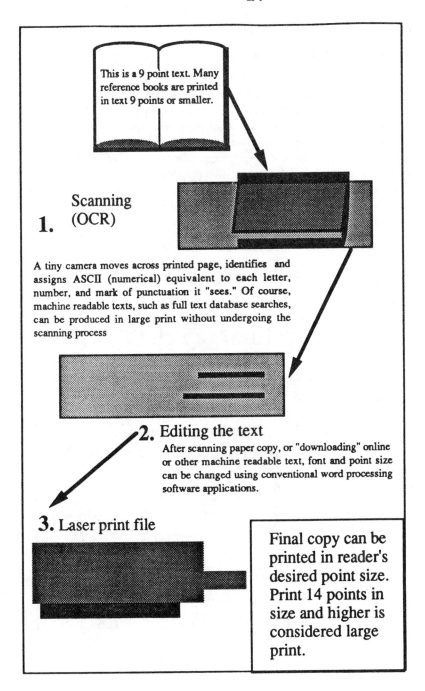

This is a 9 point text. Many reference books are printed in text 9 points or smaller.

1. Scanning (OCR)

A tiny camera moves across printed page, identifies and assigns ASCII (numerical) equivalent to each letter, number, and mark of punctuation it "sees." Of course, machine readable texts, such as full text database searches, can be produced in large print without undergoing the scanning process

2. Editing the text

After scanning paper copy, or "downloading" online or other machine readable text, font and point size can be changed using conventional word processing software applications.

3. Laser print file

Final copy can be printed in reader's desired point size. Print 14 points in size and higher is considered large print.

Figure 10. Desktop large print text production

Enlargement Technologies

Closed Circuit Television

Closed circuit television enlargement (CCTV) devices were introduced in the early 1970s, and quickly became popular reading aids for low-vision readers. Dr. Natalie Barraga's research into the use of residual vision, mentioned earlier, did much to encourage the acceptance and widespread use of this technology by people with limited vision.

CCTV devices consist of three components: a video display (television screen), a movable platform on which reading material is placed, and a video camera directed toward that platform (see figure 11). The basic CCTV configuration may be supplemented by motorized viewing tables (intended for use by readers with mobility impairments), external cameras for viewing distant objects (such as blackboards), foot pedals, or other adaptations. For

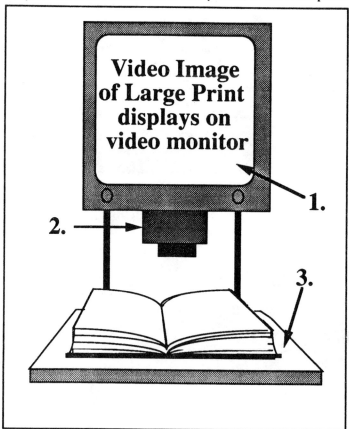

Figure 11. Closed circuit television (CCTV) components: (1) video monitor, (2) closed circuit video camera, (3) movable platform for printed materials

most libraries, the basic CCTV device will be sufficient, and will become a popular reading aid to a wide variety of library users.

The number of applications for this technology, and the potentially large audience for print enlargement, make this a likely first consideration for the library seeking to make its collections accessible to print-impaired readers. Virtually any printed material can be enlarged, with printed letters becoming as big as 4 inches or more. The largest type in large print books is no more than 24 points (1/3 inch in height), and this is not an adequate degree of enlargement for many readers with low vision. A further advantage of CCTV technology is its ability to enlarge both printed and *handwritten* material. Even pictures and graphics can be enlarged to allow independent access by readers with varying degrees of visual acuity. CCTV devices require virtually no training time; after a brief introduction the novice user can begin reading.

Just about anything that can fit under the CCTV camera can be enlarged to the individual's preferred type size. Even the cards in a catalog drawer can be magnified, unless the drawer is too tightly packed. In a recent study of the use of various adaptive technologies by library staff at the American Foundation for the Blind, head librarian Leslie Rosen pointed out the incredible versatility of CCTV technology: "Another handy discovery by a visually impaired librarian was a certain way of positioning a card catalog drawer under the CCTV camera so that a low-vision patron might enlarge the tiny print on the cards, and thus be able to select materials and carry out research independently."[22] At the AFB Library, a small wedge (very similar to a wooden door prop) is kept near the CCTV enlarger and is used by visually impaired staff and patrons to prop catalog drawers upright for enlargement by the CCTV.

If placed in the reference room, the CCTV can be used with the many very small print reference sources mentioned earlier, like the *Citation Indexes*. Some larger public libraries have strategically placed CCTV monitors throughout the library. New York Public Library's Mid-Manhattan Branch, for example, offers access to three CCTV enlargers, and these are very frequently in use by the library's many low-vision patrons. Some readers with very low vision also rely on audio output options (talking books and computers equipped with synthetic speech) for much of their extended reading. Enlarging text to the maximum size on a CCTV reading device can result in very slow reading speeds; for certain types of reading, however, patrons may prefer closed-circuit enlargement. In a reference context, for example, readers with extremely low vision might use the CCTV to scan a page of the *Library of Congress Subject Headings* before proceeding to search the online catalog which, if equipped with synthetic speech and/or a large print monitor, can be done independently.

The ability to magnify small three-dimensional objects makes the CCTV very useful to the individual who owns the device. With the CCTV, many individuals with very low vision can perform day-to-day print-related activities, such as reading appliance manuals, prescriptions and medication labels, or the cast of characters on a videocassette box.

Closed circuit television offers many options to the user. Magnification from a power of 4 to 65 produces characters ranging from 1/2 inch to over 4 inches in height. Many readers also benefit from reversed text; most CCTV devices offer positive (i.e., black characters on a white background) or negative (white characters on black) output options. Similarly, contrast and brightness may be adjusted to the individual user's needs, affording another level of control over the enlarged text image. Some CCTVs offer split-screen access to two sources simultaneously, allowing the user to read enlarged text while viewing his or her own writing or typing. The earliest CCTV devices to provide split-screen access utilized two cameras: one enlarged the reading material, and the other focused on the user's writing surface or secondary reading material. More modern CCTV devices, such as the DP11 Plus, provide enlargement of hard copy as well as access to large print characters generated by the computer.

Many CCTVs feature electronic line markers, which can be used to isolate a line of text by covering the lines above and below. This can be most useful, particularly in the reading of tabular material. Remember that the printed page must be moved on the platform from right to left in order to magnify the entire page, only a portion of which can be viewed at any one time relative to the degree of magnification employed by the system. The electronic line marker makes it easier to track one line of text, particularly when high magnification is being used.

The importance of independent access to print materials through computer technology has been emphasized throughout this text. Since the introduction of CCTV, independent research can be conducted by individuals who, in the past, would have relied on assistants for the selection of materials.

"Low-Tech" Screen Enlargement

Most reference librarians have probably encountered patrons who need help reading the characters on the online catalog or other computer display. A large group of readers in most libraries, while able to independently search the catalog, would benefit from print slightly larger than that provided by most computer monitors. One fairly inexpensive device that might benefit this population is the Compu-Lenz, a product of Able-Tech Connection (see appendix B).

The Compu-Lenz is a magnifying screen which, when attached to the computer display, enlarges characters to about twice their normal size with a minimum of distortion. The 17-inch precision crafted acrylic fresnel lens sits parallel to the 14-inch monitor at a distance of two to three inches. The lens can be attached either to the computer monitor directly or to a swivel connector that is also available from Able-Tech.

The latest Compu-Lenz model also features a nonglare screen, which eliminates interference from background lighting. An optional plastic hood seals the edges of the Compu-Lenz, filtering out any additional light that might enter the two- or three-inch space which separates the lens from the computer's screen. Unlike most of the PC-based hardware round software access products discussed below, the Compu-Lenz requires virtually no training, and will benefit a fairly large portion of the library's low-vision readership.

PC-Based Enlargement Hardware and Software

Large print computer technology, in the form of hardware or software, is used to enlarge characters on the computer monitor to a size that can be viewed with less difficulty by people with low vision. Most such adaptive devices and software programs offer a wide range of magnification, so that individual users can select the print size they are most able to read comfortably. In addition, most computer enlargement technology requires some training, and the availability of staff to provide such training should be taken into consideration by the library considering purchase of such equipment.

Screen enlargement products can be divided into two categories, based on how the user manipulates information on the screen. The system will either employ an external device (such as the DP-11 Plus's joystick) or will use the keyboard (such as LP DOS) to control which portions of the screen are enlarged. Both categories have benefits, and the choice of a system most appropriate for its application should be the result of careful consideration on the library's part. If the equipment is to be used exclusively as a large print online catalog station, for example, use of an external device, such as the DP-11 Plus might be most appropriate. Screen-enlarging software, on the other hand, has the advantage of portability. The user who is comfortable with LP DOS will be able to make use of numerous systems throughout the library simply by loading the large print software into the PC, assuming that each of these computers meets the specifications required by the software package. Librarians who are considering the purchase of large print hardware *or* software should be especially careful in noting the requirements of each system. If compatibility with existing equipment is an issue (and when is it not?), specifications of all equipment should be noted, and compatibility should be a primary concern in dealings with salespeople.

PC-based screen enlargement products intercept and reconfigure ASCII characters before they are displayed on the computer's monitor. Some such devices convert ASCII characters by enlarging pixels, and result in a jagged-edged character. Others produce smoother, sometimes rounded letter forms and other characters by completely redrawing the ASCII character before it appears on the screen.

Almost all enlargement devices and software are designed to work with specific types of monitors. For IBM and IBM-compatible PCs, there are three basic monitor options available: EGA (Enhanced Graphics Adaptor), MDA (Monochrome Display Adaptor), and CGA (Color Graphics Adaptor). CGA monitors can display a range of up to sixteen colors with enhanced clarity of characters. EGA monitors extend the range of color options from sixteen to the full palette of 256 colors. MDA monitor adaptors provide enhanced clarity to traditional, two-color monochrome displays.

Most large print computer access products were designed to work with colors, with the exception of the DP-11 Plus, a hardware device that displays text in black and white only. The DP-11 Plus utilizes the CCTV technology described earlier to provide split-screen access to both online and hard copy sources. A closed-circuit camera enlarges text on a portion of the screen, with the size of the enlargement controllable by the user. For the many libraries which have both online (for recent acquisitions) and card catalogs, the DP-11 Plus, if placed in or near the catalog room, can be used as a magnification tool for both of these important reference resources. The DP-11's control panel features a joystick, which separates screen manipulation functions from the keyboard, making the system fairly easy to master by the user unfamiliar with high-tech gadgetry. Its ability to display a full range of ASCII characters, including symbols, diacritics, etc., further extends the power of this large print computer access device.

Another split-screen enlargement device, the Optelec 20/20, offers access to hard copy as well as computer display enlargement. Magnifiying printed materials up to sixty times, the 20/20 offers the features one expects to find in a video enlargement device—contrast and brightness controls and normal and reverse image modes. A number of system options, such as a remote video camera intended for use with distant objects (blackboards, etc.), provide further alternatives for the print-impaired reader.

Similar devices are listed and briefly described in appendix B.

Screen-Access Software

One of the earliest and most popular software packages available for large print access to the computer display is PC Lens, available from Arts Computer Products (see appendix B). PC Lens requires a CGA adaptor card, described above, which affords the user some control over colors used to display text as well as special attributes of that text. Highlighted text, for example, can be displayed in a color chosen by the user. Like the speech access systems described in the previous chapter, PC Lens and other large print software products allow the user to move around the screen in what is referred to as "review mode." Using the F1 key, the user enters the review mode, and may then move around the screen using a series of control keys. Remember that, depending on the degree of magnification, only a portion of the regular display may be viewed at any one time. With magnification set at 16 power, for example, only one line may be viewed at a time. The ability to easily control what appears on the screen will, of course, greatly affect the user's reading speed.

ZoomText, another large print screen-access program, also provides magnification up to 16 power, providing very crisp, enlarged ASCII characters. Degree of magnification is easily altered using the keyboard's + and – keys. ZoomText Plus, also available from AI Squared (see appendix B), provides access to Microsoft Windows and all of the Windows applications. Navigation options include the use of the keyboard or a standard mouse. The ZoomText products are easy to learn and use, and the option of mouse-controlled navigation frees the keyboard for other uses.

Version 5.0 LP DOS, a screen enlargement product distributed in the United States by Optelec, Inc. (see appendix B), provides clear magnification of both text and graphics on IBM-compatible PCs as well as on the IBM PS/2. Like the other products mentioned so far, LP DOS allows a maximum magnification of 16 power. Version 5.0 of this popular enlargement system is completely interactive with Windows, as well as all of the major application software like WordPerfect and Lotus 1-2-3. LP DOS requires a monitor equipped with an EGA, VGA, or CGA display adaptor, and provides two modes of screen navigation. Using either the computer's keyboard or a standard mouse, users can easily control which section of the screen is viewed. LP DOS offers a variety of advanced features, but basic screen navigation commands are easy to learn and new users can begin using the software with a limited amount of training. LP DOS 5.0, when in review mode, will completely disable the synthetic speech program; however, when the synthetic speech screen-access software is in review mode, LP DOS will remain operational, continuing to track the cursor and enlarge ASCII characters.

Most screen enlargement products are designed to work in tandem with synthetic speech screen-access software. Many users with limited vision augment their use of screen enlargement with synthetic speech, which can result in increased reading speed. While most enlargement products are designed with this in mind, the consumer is advised to go beyond the vendor's literature in researching any product. The American Foundation for the Blind and other not-for-profit organizations listed in appendix A can be of assistance to the consumer seeking information on product compatibility and other issues. In fact, AFB maintains a database of users who can provide first-hand knowledge of products to individuals or institutions considering the purchase of a specific software or hardware system.

Remember also that training is an issue with large print access devices as well as with other adaptive technologies. In the next chapter, we will talk about accessible online catalogs and explore training in much greater detail. We will see that hardware and software do not, by themselves, render computers instantly accessible to our target population. The enlargement products discussed in this section require greatly varying degrees of training. An online catalog equipped with an external device that uses a joystick might provide almost instant access for the new user. Separating screen navigation functions from the keyboard by the use of an external device will in itself eliminate some confusion on the user's part. Even with the easiest and most logically designed products, however, librarians should expect any new equipment to require an investment in time for orientation and training.

Reference Services to Readers with Low Vision

It is not within the scope of this monograph to identify all of the conditions and degrees of vision loss that are collectively experienced by low-vision readers, nor is it our business to prescribe specific reading aids. In order to effectively serve the large and rapidly growing population of patrons with limited vision, however, librarians must have an understanding of the effects of low vision on the *individual reader*. Remember that, unlike blind readers, who are usually recognizable, low-vision readers are often not immediately identifiable as such. The librarian must have certain information about the patron's needs in order to assist in the selection and use of materials, and this information will probably be elicited during the course of the reference interview, assuming that the reader identifies him- or herself as visually impaired.

Like many people with learning disabilities, the low-vision reader's disability can be "invisible." But unlike patrons with learning disabilities, who can be reluctant to identify themselves as such, people with low vision are usually forthcoming with information about their disability. Furthermore, most librarians will agree that it is the rare patron who knows exactly what he or she wants, and readers with low vision are probably no exception to the rule. The reference librarian's challenge is compounded vis-à-vis patrons with limited vision by the need to understand which materials, formats, and/or technologies the reader wants or expects in addition to the "content" of the reference query.

The patron's identification of him- or herself as visually impaired is obviously intended to elicit a response. Furthermore, the statement might mean any number of things. The patron might simply be asking for assistance with something in the reference room—such as finding a call number in the catalog or on a shelf, reading an entry in an index, etc. Unless the statement is part of a request for concrete information (e.g., "I have a visual impairment. Does the library have a selection of reference books in large print?"), the librarian will have to attempt to discover what the patron's real needs are. The patron might own a CCTV enlarger he or she uses to magnify printed materials, but might need the librarian's help in retrieving a reference item, such as an article from an encyclopedia. Another patron might simply need assistance using an index, but can locate materials in the stacks, read call numbers without assistance, etc. Sometimes the person will want to find out what kinds of services are available for the visually impaired. In most cases, the librarian needs the *patron's* guidance in order to pursue the most appropriate course of action during the reference encounter.

While we never really *prescribe* reading aids, librarians can *expose* their patrons to enlargement devices and other adaptive technologies. In so doing, libraries are performing a vital service to their patrons, many of whom might not know that certain options are available. Bruce Massis, Director of Library Services at the Jewish Guild for the Blind in New York, points out that contrary to what we might expect, ophthalmologists are not always aware of the current state of adaptive technology for print-impaired readers. For some readers diagnosed with limited vision, the library can provide exposure to an array of devices that might extend their options for independent access to printed or online materials.

Librarians are further warned to proceed cautiously. Some of the technologies presented in this chapter provide us with the ability to produce high-quality materials in large print format, for example. One might expect that the patron who uses large print would prefer 20-point to 16-point type, basing this on the assumption that the larger the print, the easier it will be to read. For some readers with limited vision, those extra 4 points are not desirable, and serve only to *decrease* reading speed.

The information necessary to avoid the misuse of materials and technologies can be acquired, but this requires communication between patron and librarian. In the previous example, point size selection might be made by the reader before the printing process begins. The patron will not necessarily know his or her preferred point size, but will be able to select from a sheet of examples. A chart that illustrates point sizes (such as figure 6, but perhaps offering a complete range of sizes from 12 through 24 point) might be presented to the reader to assist in the selection of a type size that would be most comfortable for the individual.

As our knowledge of print impairment increases, so will our ability to serve our readers with disabilities. First the library has to determine which devices and services it intends to have available for its visually impaired patrons. Then the librarian must work with the individual patrons to provide the best utilization of these offerings according to the patron's specific needs.

Notes

1. Otto Hallauer, "Die Brille 100 Jahre vor und 100 Jahre nach der Erfindung der Buchdruckerkunst," in *Universitäts-Augenklinik und Augenheilanstalt Basel 1864–1914*, edited by professor Carl Mellinger (Basle, 1915), 121–39. Quoted in John Dreyfus, "The Invention of Spectacles and the Advent of Printing," in *The Library*, 6th ser. 10, no. 2 (June 1988): 104.
2. Linda Redmond, "Large Print Books and Magazines, in *Encyclopedia of Library and Information Science*, vol. 37, supp. 2 (New York: Marcel Dekker), 202.
3. Ibid., 205.
4. Torsten Andersson, "Microfiche as a Reading Aid for Partially Sighted Students," *Journal of Visual Impairment and Blindness* 74 (May 1980): 193–96.
5. Robert B. Irwin, *Classes for the Conservation of Vision*, manuscript, 1916, 1.
6. American Foundation for the Blind, *Directory of Services for Blind and Visually Impaired Persons in the United States*, 23d ed. (New York, 1988), A8.
7. Arnold Sorsby, "Blindness in the World Today," *WHO Chronicle* 21 (Sept. 1967): 369.
8. Eleanor E. Faye, *Clinical Low Vision* (Boston: Little, Brown, 1976), 8.
9. Natalie C. Barraga, "Utilization of Low Vision in Adults Who Are Severely Visually Handicapped," *New Outlook for the Blind* 70 (May 1976): 177.
10. Ibid, 58.
11. Redmond, "Large Print Books and Magazines," 202.
12. Joel A. Roth, "Low-Vision Readers," *Talking Book Topics* 31 (Sept. 1965): 140.
13. Redmond, "Large Print Books and Magazines," 205.
14. Judith Lee Palmer, "Large-Print Books: Public Library Services to Older Adults," *Educational Gerontology* 14 (1988): 220.
15. Diane Wolfe, New York Public Library for the Blind and Physically Handicapped, telephone interview with Tom McNulty, March 25, 1992.
16. Carolyn Anthony, "More Eyes on Large Print: With New Players in the Field, Older and Younger Readers Are Getting a Wider Choice of Titles and Faster Delivery of Bestsellers," *Publishers Weekly*, Jan. 25, 1991, 18–23.
17. Other early "Books for Tired Eyes" inventories included *Books for Children with Seriously Defective Vision* (New York Library Assn., 1939); *Save Your Eyes: A List of Library Books for Visually Handicapped Children* (Oregon State Library, 1950); and *Easy On The Eyes* (Cleveland Public Library, 1957).
18. New York Public Library, *Large Print Book Project: A Report* (New York, 1969), 23.
19. Ibid.
20. As of April 24, 1992.
21. Bruce Massis, librarian, Jewish Guild for the Blind, telephone interview with Tom McNulty, April 26, 1992.
22. Leslie Rosen, "Enabling Blind and Visually Impaired Library Users: InMagic and Adaptive Technologies," *Library Hi Tech* 9 (1991): 55.

Chapter Six

Programs and Services

In our discussions of braille, audio, and large print, we have touched upon several issues of historical concern as well as some current trends in library applications of technology and accessible text formats. In the following pages, we will describe the many ways in which the new technologies can be used to fully integrate the print-impaired reader into the mainstream library environment, offering suggestions for the development of both a talking computerized card catalog and hi-tech resource center. We conclude with the presentation of two models, one a high-tech, highly funded academic library, the other a moderate size, moderately funded public facility.

Access Methods

By the end of the nineteenth century, when the public library movement was well underway and the American Library Association was established as the national forum for librarians' concerns on a variety of issues, several large public libraries were already providing service and materials to people with disabilities. A 1904 *Public Libraries* report indicated that "at least eighteen public libraries in large cities are serving blind readers."[1] With relatively few accessible texts available for use by print-impaired patrons, public library programming for blind readers at the turn of the century consisted of readings, recitals, lectures, gallery visits, and other similar activities. But by 1904, "more than ninety percent of books lent by libraries for the blind were requested by mail or telephone, and practically all were sent out through the post office."[2] With the passage of legislation governing postage-free mailing of reading materials for the blind, the nature of library service to patrons with disabilities quickly shifted from planned programming to a kind of correspondence service.

While those early library-sponsored events for blind patrons might be seen as attempts at mainstreaming the visually impaired reader into the library, the primary service of most libraries, particularly public libraries, was then and is now the provision of materials on loan. At the turn of the century, however, braille was still relatively new in the United States, and consequently there were very few embossed titles available for loan. This situation was further complicated by the number of different embossing systems in use until 1918, when braille was accepted as the standard by the American Association of Workers for the Blind. Oral readings, both for groups and individuals, were important because of the dearth of materials available to the print-impaired population.

The progress made in the production of braille texts, as well as the introduction of postage-free circulation of embossed texts for use by the blind, did much to encourage independence among print-impaired readers. Patrons soon discovered that there was little reason to actually visit the library since materials could be ordered by mail or by phone and then delivered to them in their homes. Thus, the National Library Service, which has played a central role in virtually all aspects of library service to patrons with disabilities, evolved into an enormous national "books by mail" service. The NLS continues to conduct most of its transactions through the mail, but in many ways the new technologies and accessible text formats described in the previous chapters are changing the role of libraries from mail-order book services to environments that are compatible with disabled patrons.

A prerequisite to any patron's effective use of all the library's resources is independent access to reference tools—notably, the catalog(s). Until recently, blind and visually impaired library users had to rely almost exclusively on librarians or readers to assist them in their selection of materials. Few libraries outside the NLS network offered texts in formats that were accessible to print-impaired individuals; at best, the typical public library might have had a selection of large type books. Blind and low-vision patrons of public, academic, and other types of libraries required assistance not only in searching the catalogs, but in reading the texts themselves. Thus, the need for assistance did not end once materials were identified and located; the services of readers were required by blind patrons in all other aspects of reading and research.

We have seen how microcomputer technology has dramatically increased the options available to the print-impaired reader in search of accessible texts. High technology is not in itself sufficient to render libraries accessible to people with disabilities. In our discussion of services, outreach, and training, the importance of an overall program will be stressed. The patron who can independently search the online catalog may still need assistance in retrieving materials from the library's stacks, photocopying or scanning books and periodicals, etc. Similarly, few librarys' holdings are completely accessible online. Most online catalogs represent but a portion of the library's holdings and are supplemented by traditional card catalogs. Print-impaired readers still need assistance in using such print-based tools. The accessible library will provide staff to assist in these important aspects of library service.

The Online Catalog

Most online catalogs are designed for use by patrons with little or no experience with computers. Simple author, title, or subject searches of the library's holdings are generally as easy as checking one's balance at an automatic teller machine. Where more complicated search strategies are employed (Boolean searching, etc.), the patron is usually guided by menus and online help screens. Once a terminal has been equipped with an adaptive screen-access system, these same menus and help screens can guide blind, visually impaired, and learning-disabled patrons through any number of complex searches. The system script need not be modified as efforts to simplify access techniques can be made via the adaptive system itself. Indeed, the amount of training required to enable the print-impaired user to gain proficiency with this system should be only slightly greater than that required to facilitate the sighted patron's use of the online catalog. Clearly, the need for any increased training will be dependent upon the print-impaired patron's familiarity with the access system in use. Under these circumstances, however, it will not be incumbent upon the library to ensure the blind or visually impaired user's proficiency with the screen-access system independent of the OPAC application itself. As mentioned earlier, modifications may be made to the access system's standard configuration in order to facilitate use of the library-specific script. Users need not, therefore, master the access system in its entirety in order to search the catalog independently.

Interface Options

Each of the computer access technologies presented in the previous chapters can be used to render the library's online catalog and other electronic information sources accessible. The catalog equipped with a soft braille device is accessible to any braille reader, including those who are both deaf and blind. The synthetic speech screen-access software described in chapter 4 can be used to convert the library's OPAC into a talking system, rendering the system accessible to patrons with visual and/or learning disabilities. The OPAC interfaced with any of the large print peripherals described in the previous chapter will extend access to readers with low vision, including the rapidly growing elderly population.

Despite the quality and rapidly declining prices of adaptive computer products, surprisingly few libraries are exploiting any of these new technologies to the benefit of their disabled readership. The library literature indicates a strong interest by librarians in the provision of online service to readers with disabilities, but there seems to be some confusion as to what a talking OPAC terminal should actually do.

As effective use of most of the adaptive devices described in the previous chapters requires a considerable amount of training and practice, there simply is no user-friendly interface available that will render computerized catalogs as instantly accessible to the blind and visually impaired reader as they are to the sighted population. This situation is compounded by the number and variety of screen-access products on the market. Here the burden is greatest on the print-impaired individual who wants access to a number of libraries and the vast array of electronic sources available to other library users. Most sighted people can move from a GEAC terminal to an Innopac online catalog with few problems. If the talking version of the GEAC catalog uses Artic as its screen-access system, and the Innopac employs Vert software, the blind person who wants that same level of independent access must learn enough about both adaptive devices to navigate the screens of each system effectively.

The problem has been articulated by Lana Dixon, reference librarian at the University of Tennessee, Knoxville (UTK). In her article on the provision of academic library services to patrons with disabilities, she points out the discrepancy between the existing technology and the needs of visually impaired readers:

> A talking catalog is not created simply by attaching a voice synthesizer. The GEAC system at UTK requires the user to move through several screens to arrive at the bibliographic citation that identifies call number, location, and status. A sighted user rapidly views the screens and pinpoints pertinent information. A visually impaired user needs the same ability, and software must be written to control which portions of the screen are read. Adapting any software requires the cooperation and participation of the catalog vendor. Convincing a catalog vendor to place this type of project high on the list of development priorities could well be the most daunting aspect of equipping a catalog with voice output.[3]

We would submit that since relying upon third-party solutions may not be feasible, libraries will need to take advantage of the configuration options provided with most speech-based screen-access systems to render their online catalogs fully accessible to print-impaired users.[4] If the online catalog cannot be made to conform to the needs of its print-impaired users, the screen-access device can be modified to provide a friendlier interface to the OPAC. And again, users need not be trained in all the nuances of a particular access device in order to begin using the online catalog independently.

Remote access to a growing number of information sources is, of course, one option available to the visually impaired computer user. Since few users who are not dedicated computerphiles will set out to learn the ins and outs of all the available screen-access systems, most blind and visually impaired patrons will have strong preferences regarding one or another access system. As an analogy, sighted people might consider their own computer use. Most people know one or two word-processing programs, perhaps WordPerfect for IBM and compatibles or Microsoft Word for MacIntosh computers. It is unlikely that anyone would learn an entirely new system in order to access one computer terminal if access were already possible somewhere else. Many print-impaired users will understandably prefer to access online services from their home computers via modem. But remote access does not encourage the mainstream integration of blind, visually impaired, and learning-disabled patrons. Remote computer access is little more than a hi-tech version of the "books by mail" service.

In chapter 4, we were introduced to the power and complexity of various synthetic speech systems. Before selecting any equipment, librarians are urged to obtain the advice of vision rehabilitation professionals. Some people are put off by the unnatural sound of many synthetic speech programs, and might consequently make an unwise decision in the selection of equipment. Input from users should also be encouraged. Many visually impaired individuals have experience with computers, and can educate the librarian in the pros and cons of various systems.

Technical assistance is generously provided by most of the associations identified in appendix A. The National Technology Center at the American Foundation for the Blind can be particularly informative in this regard. Regular feature articles in AFB's *Journal of Visual Impairment and Blindness (JVIB)*, as well as the Technology Center's "Random Access" column, identify, evaluate, and sometimes compare adaptive technology software and hardware products. *JVIB* is indexed in its entirety by ERIC, and is an excellent source of information on a variety of disabilities as well as library science literature on service to patrons with disabilities. Librarians who may be contemplating the purchase of screen-access equipment for their online catalogs should further consider the availability of staff to provide training and user support.

Not surprisingly, most of the library literature on talking online catalogs has been generated by academic librarians. Most larger academic libraries have a captive audience of disabled patrons who have a serious interest in learning the skills required for independent access to the library's online catalog and other systems. Disabled college students must have either independent or reader-assisted access to the library's catalogs in order to effectively pursue a higher education. Many academic communities subsidize students' use of readers and/or provide training in the use of adaptive technology. Since the question of just who is responsible for training disabled readers in the use of technology tends to be a difficult issue to resolve, academic librarians may wish to contact the disabled student center at their colleges in order to determine whether any provision is made for training and ongoing user support. According to a recent survey of academic and research library programs of services to patrons with disabilities, the vast majority of respondents indicate that disabled readers' services are handled by reference department staff.[5]

The Accessible Catalog

In order to maximize the user-friendliness of an online catalog equipped with synthetic speech output, a number of system adaptations can be made to assist the user in navigating screens that were designed with sighted users in mind. While we agree with Lana Dixon that "a talking catalog is not created simply by attaching a voice synthesizer," it is our belief that the powerful customization capabilities of most synthetic speech screen-access systems can be used to render the OPAC extremely user-friendly.

Recall that configuration files are routinely written to handle the particular features of programs such as WordPerfect, dBase, and Lotus 1-2-3; generating configuration files and user-definable dictionaries that are designed for use with a particular OPAC script is no more difficult than generating such files for use with standard business applications. The purpose of any synthetic speech screen-access device is to enable users to operate effectively within the bounds of a particular application. Thus, flexibility is inherent in any high-quality access system. Some degree of training with both the access system and its relationship to the online catalog will naturally be required before the user will be able to conduct bibliographic searches independently. Taking New York University's (NYU) GEAC online catalog, BobCat, as our example, we will offer configuration options and training suggestions to help users maximize their efficiency with several screens they will encounter.

Talking BobCat

BobCat (short for Bobst Catalog), is Bobst Library's online catalog. This GEAC system contains records for approximately one-third of the library's holdings. In addition to Bobst Library, several other libraries within the NYU Library system are represented in the online catalog. As of May 1992, BobCat contained close to one million bibliographic records.

Although the library's dedicated Bobcat terminals are not actual PCs, we would submit that workstations designated for use by blind, visually impaired, and learning-disabled users be standalone units having network access to the online catalog. The reasons for this particular configuration are manifold. Whether the accessible unit is to be equipped with screen magnification or synthetic speech software or both, the system must be immediately accessible. That is, the access software should boot with the PC or be easily selected from a menu before any applications software, including the OPAC script, is loaded. The adaptive software can be stored on the network file server or locally on a hard disk, but it must be easily invoked by blind, visually impaired, and learning-disabled users. Moreover, the GEAC hardware is unusual in that the keyboard is outfitted with several unfamiliar keys. For example, a large red key labeled "Send" replaces the traditional "Enter" key. Because most synthetic speech programs will not recognize this key (as well as several others), the terminal equipped with synthetic speech output should not employ the GEAC keyboard, but a standard 101 keyboard. In this way, input conflicts between the application and the access device are minimized as is the potential for user disorientation.

Figures 12 through 18 show the first seven screens encountered by the novice conducting a title search on BobCat. Note that the menu of search options does not appear until the third screen. This information is preceded by an introductory screen and a "news" screen, which is updated periodically. The options presented on the introductory screen (see figure 12), which can be invoked at any time, are easily selected on dedicated BobCat terminals by hitting one of eight designated function keys. Users of Talking BobCat have the same options, but must enter each command as a text string. In order to return to the previous screen, for example, the user would type the words PREVIOUS SCREEN, followed by Enter.

We have seen the benefits of such text-based systems in our discussion of synthetic speech screen-access in chapter 4. Fortunately, Bobcat employs no graphics and, in fact, makes use of a command line so that, in general,

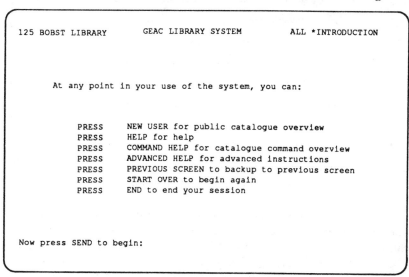

```
  125 BOBST LIBRARY        GEAC LIBRARY SYSTEM          ALL *INTRODUCTION



        At any point in your use of the system, you can:


             PRESS      NEW USER for public catalogue overview
             PRESS      HELP for help
             PRESS      COMMAND HELP for catalogue command overview
             PRESS      ADVANCED HELP for advanced instructions
             PRESS      PREVIOUS SCREEN to backup to previous screen
             PRESS      START OVER to begin again
             PRESS      END to end your session



  Now press SEND to begin:
```

Figure 12. BobCat introduction screen

```
125 BOBST LIBRARY       GEAC LIBRARY SYSTEM        ALL *INTRODUCTION


                         WELCOME TO BOBCAT!

BobCat lists over 940,000 catalog records, including all material purchased
  after 1973 and many earlier items. Please check the card catalog for:
              *pre-1973 materials NOT found in BobCat, and
              *pre-1985 materials written in non-Roman scripts.


        *** TRY OUT BOBCAT'S NEW FEATURE - BOOLEAN SEARCHING ***
   Search any combination of key words from titles, subjects, or authors.
Select BOL from BobCat's main menu, then  MOR for on-screen instructions.

          NYUNET users: Type HELP <CR> for special instructions
          New BobCat Users: Press the NEW USER function key (F7)

             Type END to end your BobCat session.



Press SEND to continue
```

Figure 13. BobCat News screen

```
125 BOBST LIBRARY        GEAC LIBRARY SYSTEM         ALL *CHOOSE SEARCH


What type of search do you wish to do?

        1. TIL  - Title, journal title, series title, etc.

        2. AUT  - Author, illustrator, editor, organization, etc.

        3. A-T  - Combination of author and title.

        4. SUB  - Subject heading assigned by library.

        5. NUM  - Call number, ISBN, ISSN, etc.

        6. BOL  - Boolean search on title, author and subject

        7. LIM  - Limit your search to a portion of the catalogue.


Enter number or code: 1                          Then press SEND
```

Figure 14. BobCat main menu

the system design lends itself well to use by blind and visually impaired users. As we move from screen to screen, the cursor remains on the command line, and the user's options are always enumerated on the lines just above this command line (see figure 18). As information scrolls across the screen, users may have difficulty interpreting options, prompts, and specific bibliographic data. However, once the screen stabilizes, users may enter the

```
125 BOBST LIBRARY          GEAC LIBRARY SYSTEM          ALL *TITLE SEARCH



        Start at the beginning of the title and enter as many

        words of the title as you know below.




        EX.:  Wuthering Heights

        EX.:  How to Succeed in Business Without





   Enter title:Wuthering Heights                       Then press SEND
```

Figure 15. BobCat title search screen

```
125 BOBST LIBRARY          GEAC LIBRARY SYSTEM          ALL *CHOOSE SEARCH


     Your title: Wuthering Heights                  matches    9 titles

                                                     No of citations
                                                     in entire catalog


     1 Wuthering Heights /                                        14
     2 Wuthering Heights: an anthology of criticism               1
     3 Wuthering Heights: an authoritative text with essays in criti> 2
     4 Wuthering Heights: authoritative text, backgrounds, criticism/ 1
     5 Wuthering Heights: complete, authoritative text with biograph> 1
     6 Wuthering Heights (Emily Bronte)                            1
     7 Wuthering Heights [sound recording] /                       1
     8 Wuthering Heights: text, sources, criticism                 1
     9 Wuthering Heights [videorecording] /                        1


     Enter number or code                            Then press SEND
```

Figure 16. BobCat index screen

review mode or use the adaptive device's dedicated cursor to browse
through the information on the video display, picking out items of interest
in much the same way sighted users do.

When designing a speech-based accessible OPAC, technicians will want
to make use of the adaptive device's windowing capabilities to enhance the
speed with which end users will be able to navigate the screen. We have
already described the benefits of a command line environment, but notice

```
 125 BOBST LIBRARY        GEAC LIBRARY SYSTEM        ALL *TITLE SEARCH

                                                   has   14 citations
      This title:  Wuthering Heights /             in entire catalog

 Ref #   Author              Title                    Date
     1   Bronte, Emily, 1818-1848.   Wuthering Heights /    1956
     2   Bronte, Emily, 1818-1848.   Wuthering Heights /    1976
     3   Bronte, Emily, 1818-1848.   Wuthering Heights /    1980
     4   Bronte, Emily, 1818-1848    Wutherin Heights /     1988
     5   Bronte, Emily Jane, 1818-1848.  Wuthering heights /  1907
     6   Bronte, Emily Jane, 1818-1848   Wuthering Heights.   1907
     7   Bronte, Emily Jane, 1818-1848.  Wuthering heights.   1929
     8   Bronte, Emily Jane, 1818-1848   Wuthering Heights.   1940
     9   Bronte, Emily Jane, 1818-1848.  Wuthering Heights.   1950
    10   Bronte, Emily Jane, 1818-1848.  Wuthering Heights.   1950
    11   Bronte, Emily Jane, 1818-1848.  Wuthering Heights    1986

 Type a number to see associate information -OR-

    IND - see list of heading        FOR - move forward in this list
    CAT - begin a new search

    Enter number or code                      Then press SEND
```

Figure 17. BobCat citation screen

```
 125 BOBST LIBRARY        GEAC LIBRARY SYSTEM        ALL *CHOOSE SEARCH


 AUTHOR   Bronte, Emily, 1818-1848.
 TITLE:  Wuthering Heights / Emily Bronte; edited by Hilda Marsden and Ia>
 IMPRINT: Oxford : Clarendon Press, 1976.

    Location                      Cpy
                                   #        Status

 BOBST /BSTACK
      Call Number: PR4172.W7x 1976            Overdue
                                   1

 BOBST /BSTACK
      Call Number: PR4172.W7x 1976   2        In Library

 ┌──────────────────────────────────────────────────────────────────┐
 │ BRF - see locations and call numbers    FUL - see complete citation │
 │ CIT - return to your citation list      IND - see list of headings  │
 │ FOR - see next citation in list         BAC - see previous citation │
 │ CAt - begin a new search                CMD - see additional commands│
 └──────────────────────────────────────────────────────────────────┘

    Enter code                               Then press SEND
```

*Figure 18. BobCat citation screen—brief display. Commands in box
at bottom of screen represent user's options.*

that the Bobcat command line consistently appears on line 23 of the display.
This consistency enables the creation of a window whose boundaries will
be set to line 23, columns 1 through 80. This window is then assigned to a
program-specific hot key (e.g., Alt 1) so that users may easily access the
information on line 23 at any time during the session. Generally speaking,
all relevant information begins at approximately line 3 in the Bobcat

display; i.e., the words, "171 Bobst Library—GEAC Library System" continuously appear at the top of each new screen. As this information is not necessary for the user, it can be removed from the primary viewing window or, in the alternative, prevented from being verbalized within access systems that have either a "create special dictionary" or "ignore text string" function. In many ways, the user-definable dictionary option available with most synthetic speech access systems will be as helpful in providing a friendly interface to the online catalog as is the ability to create windows. Where windows provide users with direct access to important areas of the screen, the user-definable dictionary can be crucial to the proper comprehension of the information found in those windows.

Consider figure 14: This is the first screen in which the user encounters the menu of search options. Note that the commands are text strings that must be entered on the command line—TIL for a title search, AUT for an author search, BOL for a Boolean search, etc. The novice synthetic speech user may have some difficulty interpreting the system's peculiar pronunciation of the codes and may consequently enter inappropriate text. The code for a Boolean search might be entered as BAL or BUL or even BOOL by the inexperienced user. Several unsuccessful attempts could result in considerable frustration. Using the access system's review cursor, one could obtain a character by character reading of the code but even this requires a fair bit of proficiency with the access system itself. A user-definable dictionary could, however, virtually eliminate this type of confusion. The dictionary would be set to verbalize the code BOL as B O L; AUT becomes A U T; and TIL is pronounced as T I L, etc. These dictionaries should be loaded along with the specific configuration file that is to be used with the OPAC.

Training

While the configuration and dictionary files described above will surely facilitate the individual end user's independent operation of the OPAC, virtually all users will require some degree of training. Even those who are proficient with the access system in use will need to be informed of the presence of special windows and other program-specific configurations. Users of screen-enlarging hard- and software will generally require less instruction in the use of the access system as no provision need be made for special windows or dictionaries. The information on the screen is simply magnified so that browsing the video display is not significantly different for most low-vision patrons. Since the magnification will, in some cases, result in a reduction in the amount of text that can be displayed on a given screen, various navigation techniques will need to be demonstrated nonetheless. We would suggest that librarians or other staff who may be employed to train print-impaired patrons in the use of the accessible online catalog limit the demonstration and discussion of the access system to only those aspects that relate specifically to the use of the catalog. Doing so will not only minimize user confusion but, more importantly, will allow the focus of the training session to be geared toward specific search strategies. Many blind and visually impaired users will have had little or no prior experience with Library of Congress subject headings, for example, and will ultimately benefit more from the librarian's knowledge in this area; once the basics of the screen-access system have been acquired, users will gain proficiency only through practice. If subject searches are consistently unsuccessful, the user may be understandably disinclined to continue in the activities that are necessary for a proficient use of both the access system and the catalog.

As previously recommended, training materials should be produced in a variety of accessible text formats. These materials should cover not only the proper use of the access system or systems but should include tutorials designed to assist all new users (disabled or not) in acquiring advanced research skills. As mentioned in chapter 4, the interactive nature of such tutorials generally leads to hard copy rather than to electronic formats. For the blind, visually impaired, or learning-disabled user, "hard copy" translates to braille, large-print, and/or audiocassette. Quick reference guides and command summaries produced in these formats may also benefit print-impaired users. For those who may already be skilled computer users, the availability of reference materials and user's guides in machine-readable format is certainly an option although we would argue that this format is not necessarily well-suited to tutorials and practice exercises.

Staffing

As the development of a user-friendly accessible catalog will require some degree of proficiency with the access system or systems to be used, libraries may wish to hire an adaptive technology specialist to initiate the project. Once the system has been properly configured, however, matters of routine maintenance might easily be attended to by either the library's local area network (LAN) administrator, specially trained librarian, or another member of the staff who has had experience with microprocessing technology. Indeed, in an academic environment, a workstudy student from the computer science or vocational rehabilitation department might be employed on a part-time basis to oversee both equipment maintenance and user support. We would, however, urge that a professional librarian either conduct or supervise all catalog training.

Library Programs for Patrons with Disabilities

In the following section, we present models of two library centers for services to disabled readers, beginning with a state-of-the-art academic library adaptive technology center. Designed for use not only by the library's own patrons with disabilities, but also as a research and demonstration center for various academic departments including vocational counseling, special education, and other rehabilitation-related fields, this configuration is possible only with the commitment of considerable financial support from public, private, and university sources. Our second proposal is designed for a public library working with a modest budget. Access is provided to a limited number of adaptive devices, and more attention is given to programming and outreach services, particularly to the community's considerable elderly population. Each proposal includes a description of the target audience, inventory of equipment, and the all-important statement of mission.

Academic Library Center

Institution: Large State University
Student Body: 25,000
Disabled Population: 305, of which:
    190 learning disabled
    50 visually impaired (including 8 totally blind)
    35 mobility impairments
    30 deaf
Note: numbers represent students, staff, and faculty registered for services with Large State University's Center for Access; it is believed that approximately twice as many "undeclared" learning-disabled and low-vision readers actually use the library and will benefit from certain adaptations of automated services.

Serving a student body of 25,000, Large State University Library houses approximately 1.25 million items. The library has a longstanding commitment to serving its disabled clientele, which has been rewarded by increased state funding as well as dontations of equipment and financial assistance from corporations and individuals. Since the passage of Section 504 of the Rehabilitation Act of 1973, the university's Section 504 committee, which is composed of staff, students, faculty, and administrators, has been charged with finding ways in which the university can be made more accessible to people with a variety of disabilities.

Services for students, faculty, and staff with disabilities are coordinated by the university's Center for Access, formerly the Center for Disabled Students. Center for Access staff provide disabled clients with everything from personal and vocational counseling to training in the use of adaptive computer equipment. Professional counseling staff include specialists in vision, deafness, and learning disabilities. The center has a philosophy of training for independence and self-advocacy.

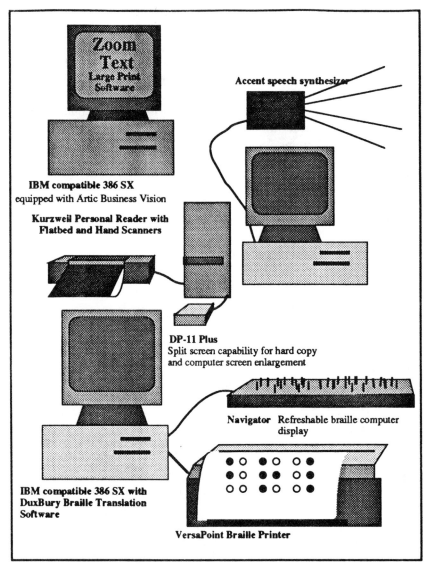

Figure 19. Technology configuration—Large Academic Library

When plans were announced for the construction of a new university library, planning began at once for the new library's Center for Readers with Disabilities. In its old quarters, the library's adaptive computer technology was located in a room much too small to handle the amount of use it was getting; indeed, the library's inventory of adaptive devices could not increase, even though sources of funding had been secured, because of the lack of space available for expansion.

The university's Section 504 committee was involved in every stage of planning the new facility. Input from physically challenged individuals guided architects in the placement of high-use study and conference rooms. Physical accessibility guidelines established under the recently passed Americans with Disabilities Act were studied and adhered to in all aspects of the design of the new facility.[6]

Students with visual impairments and/or learning disabilities were similarly polled, and their responses were taken into consideration in the selection of reading aids. Surprisingly, almost every available screen-access package was suggested for purchase by one or more of the university's 240 visually impaired and learning-disabled students. Many students have their own personal computers equipped with synthetic speech output and/or large print software or hardware devices. It soon became obvious that the center would have to provide access for a wide range of adaptive software and hardware to appeal to the majority of disabled students registered for services.

The university was able to secure state funding for the purchase of several adaptive devices because of its willingness to provide demonstrations of its equipment and limited training for its use to clients referred by the state's Office for Vocational Rehabilitation. Visually impaired clients who might benefit from screen-reading software, hardware, and other adaptive devices are allowed to use the facilities at Large State University before selecting the devices with which they are most comfortable.

Academic departments within the university can similarly schedule time in the center to introduce their students to the variety of devices available for people with disabilities. A university-wide announcement of the new center's comprehensive facilities generated interest from diverse departments. Occupational therapy, rehabilitation counseling, and special education faculty expressed an interest in the facility. Surprisingly, several business school faculty also asked if they and their classes could be given a demonstration of the center's facilities.

The configuration of adaptive devices described in the following proposal offers a complete range of accessible formats and computer output options, including braille, audiotape, synthetic speech, and large print. Included in the proposal is the center's mission statement, plan for training and instruction, and equipment inventory. Finally, figure 19 presents a schematic diagram of the center's technology configuration.

Mission Statement

Large State University has a longstanding commitment to providing service for disabled readers, and the library has played a central role in the continued development of such services through the introduction of adaptive computer technologies, reference assistance in the form of individual consultations, and specialized bibliographic instruction sessions.

Working closely with the university's Center for Access as well as with other institutions of higher education in the area, the library keeps itself informed of new developments in access technologies and services and makes every attempt to use existing technology to its fullest.

The Center for Readers with Disabilities is intended primarily for Large State University students, but serves secondarily as a "demonstration center" for various academic departments within the university as well as for the state Office for Vocational Rehabilitation. With the opening of the new university library, the Center hopes to expand its role as a demonstration center, to be used not only by students in rehabilitation fields, but also by such diverse departments as linguistics, computer science, and business administration.

Training and Instruction

Access to staff-assisted training in the use of the Center's adaptive technology is provided by one part-time reference librarian who supervises two student interns from the university's Department of Rehabilitation Counseling. Small group sessions, scheduled at the beginning of each semester, are required of all new students, faculty, and staff registered for services with the University's Center for Access. In these general orientations, new library users are introduced to a variety of adaptive devices and services offered by the library, as well as training in the use of the library's online catalog and other electronic information sources.

Individual user training sessions are scheduled by the reference librarian who oversees the adaptive technology center. In these individual sessions, students are introduced to a variety of adaptive devices and receive in-depth training in searching the online catalog and other electronic information sources. A noncredit elective course in library research rounds out the list of bibliographic instruction activities offered by the library. In this class, research techniques, advanced training in the use of the online catalog and other electronic information sources, and assistance with conducting course-related research is provided.

The university employs one part-time staff member who retrieves materials from the stacks and photocopies and scans reserve readings, periodicals, etc. Requests for materials are submitted to the part-time disabled students assistant, who retrieves materials within a two-day turnaround time.

Equipment Inventory

Located in the library's computing center, the new Center for Readers with Disabilities provides access to all of the resources available on the library's local area network, as well as diverse services and software available on the university mainframe. Access is provided to a number of bibliographic databases, including the library's online catalog, RLIN, and

Dialog, as well as popular software applications including WordPerfect, dBase, and Lotus 1-2-3.

Three IBM 386 SX personal computers, located in a separate room adjacent to the library computing center, have been reserved for the use of disabled readers. The following adaptive devices and software packages provide braille, large print, and audio access to the wealth of print and electronic information sources offered by the library. Most products have been described in the preceding chapters, and all are listed and described in appendix B.

Reading Machine/Optical Character Recognition
Kurzweil Personal Reader—stand-alone unit, featuring both flatbed and handheld scanners
Arkenstone Reader—scanner that converts standard printed text to ASCII text files

Synthetic Speech Software and Hardware
Accent Speech Synthesizer
Artic BusinessVision
VERT Plus
Vocal-eyes

Braille
Duxbury Braille Translator—software that converts grade 1 to contracted, grade 2 braille
VersaPoint Braille Embosser—braille printer; networked to all three PCs in the Center, provides braille hard copy output from a variety of on-line and applications programs
Navigator—refreshable braille computer display

Low-Vision Reading Aids
DP-11 Plus—provides split-screen access to both hard copy (using closed-circuit television technology) and computer display
Zoomtext—PC-based screen-enlargement software
Laser printer with font software—produces high-quality large print hard copy in user's choice of typeface and point size

Public Library Adaptive Technology Center

Population Served: 30,000
Disabled Population: unknown

With a population of approximately 30,000, the Public Library of this small city houses approximately 90,000 volumes, and maintains subscriptions to approximately 340 periodicals. The library is staffed by four professional librarians and seven full-time support staff.

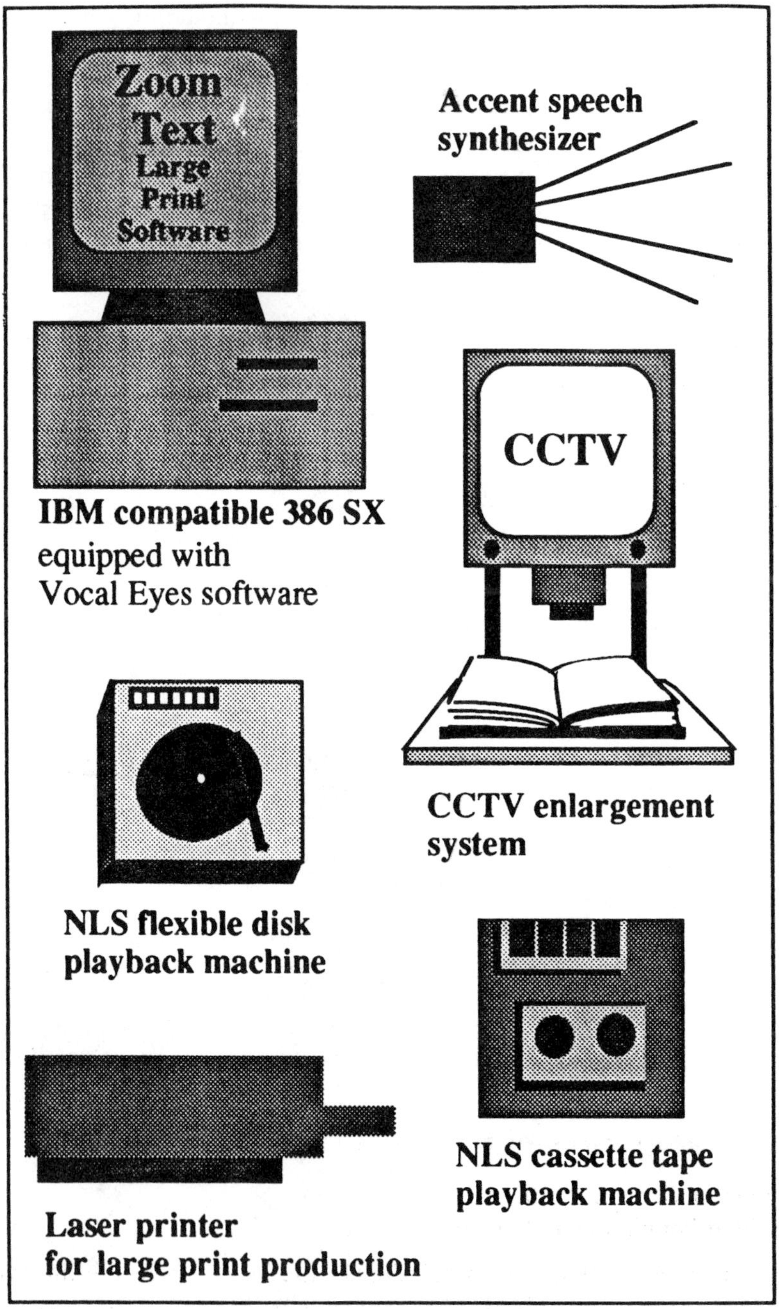

Figure 20. Technology configuration—medium-sized public library

Statistics on readers with print impairments are difficult to collect. Many elderly patrons request large type reading materials, and the library has made an attempt to acquire popular titles in this format. It is believed, however, that a great many patrons do not use the library because they are unaware of the services and facilities available. Recent outreach attempts have included visits by librarians to nursing homes, and scheduled readings in the library.

The library subscribes to *Talking Books Topics*, *Braille Books*, *Volunteers Who Produce Books*, and a number of other NLS publications. The library has also recently acquired playback equipment from the National Library Service, and librarians are available to assists patrons in applying for service as well as in the selection of materials from NLS.

In response to increased use of the center by school-aged children with a variety of disabilities, the children's librarian has established a working relationship with teachers in the local school's special education department. These teachers have provided staff training sessions in the nature of learning disabilities, and continue to work with the children's librarian on the after-school program. The homework clinic, part of the library's after-school program, has been expanded to include services for the print-impaired and is advertised through local news media and through P.T.A. announcements.

Mission Statement

This midsized public library serves a growing population of elderly readers as well as school-age children with both visual and learning disabilities. The library has made an attempt to promote service to its print-impaired readership and hopes that the new adaptive technology will serve to bring previously underserved disabled clientele into the library.

Readers with special needs are encouraged to speak with one of the reference librarians and are assured that their consultations will be confidential. Staff members can assist disabled readers in any number of ways. Training in the use of on-site adaptive technology can be scheduled through the reference department. The library also acts as an information and referral center, assisting patrons in the selection of reading materials in accessible formats within the library as well as through the National Library Service. The library maintains a collection of reading materials in large print on a variety of disabilities, as well as vertical file materials from a number of organizations concerned with people with disabilities.

The library maintains a roster of volunteer readers and other service providers and considers this an important aspect of its information and referral service. Volunteer readers work with residents of several nursing homes and provide scheduled readings for groups as well as individually arranged readings on the library premises.

Training and Instruction

Responsibility for training interested patrons in the use of adaptive technology is divided between two librarians—the children's librarian and one adult reference librarian. Prospective users *must* schedule an orientation session before being allowed access to any equipment in the adaptive technology center. Depending on the adaptive device under consideration, training may take as little as ten minutes (in the case of a CCTV enlarger), or might require several sessions of one hour each (in the case of screen-access synthetic speech).

Equipment Inventory

1 PC (IBM Compatible 386 SX)
Vocal-eyes screen-access software
Accent external speech synthesizer
ZoomText large print computer access software
Vantage CCD (closed-circuit television enlargement)
NLS cassette tape playback machine
NLS flexible disk playback machine

The library's laser printer can be scheduled for production of reading
materials in large print.

Notes

1. "What Some Libraries Are Doing for the Blind," *Public Libraries* 9 (April 1904): 150-62.
2. *That All May Read: Library Service for the Blind and Physically Handicapped* (Washington, D.C.: Library of Congress, National Library Service for the Blind and Physically Handicapped, 1983), 7.
3. Lana S. Dixon. "The Visually Impaired and the Academic Library," *College & Research Libraries News* 51 (July/Aug. 1990): 637-38.
4. See the section entitled Selection Criteria in chapter 4 for a complete discussion of program-specific configuration options.
5. *Library Service for Persons with Disabilities: SPEC Kit 176* (Washington, D.C.: Systems and Procedures Exchange Center, OMS, Association of College and Research Libraries, July/Aug 1991), 7.
6. See *Americans with Disabilities Act Handbook* (Washington, D.C.: Equal Employment Opportunity Commission and the Department of Justice).

Appendix A

Agencies and Associations

Agencies and Publishers: Visual Impairment

American Council of the Blind
1155 15th St., NW, Ste. 720
Washington, DC 20005
(202) 467-5081
Serves as a national information clearinghouse on blindness and visual impairment. Provides information, acts as advocacy and advisory group in legislative matters at all levels.

American Foundation for the Blind (AFB)
15 West 16th St.
New York, NY 10011
(212) 620-2000
Not-for-profit organization concerned with welfare of the blind and visually impaired. Publishes the multidisciplinary *Journal of Visual Impairment and Blindness*, which includes research articles on psychological, educational, legislative, and medical aspects of blindness and visual impairment. Also publishes and updates, on an irregular basis, *AFB Directory of Services for Blind and Visually Impaired Persons in the U.S.* AFB conducts research, develops and sells assistive products for the blind, and maintains both a national technology center and a research level library on blindness and visual impairment.

American Printing House for the Blind (APH)
1839 Frankfort Ave.
P.O. Box 6085
Louisville, KY 40206
(502) 895-2405

Founded in 1858, APH received federal funds for the provision of educational materials in three accessible media (braille, large type, and recorded). Manufactures, sells, and repairs Library of Congress four-track format recording equipment. Maintains a 3500- volume library. Produces an annual catalog and offers online access to APH-CARL, the complete catalog of APH offerings.

Associated Services for the Blind
919 Walnut St.
Philadelphia, PA 19107
(215) 667-0600
Produces braille and large print books, under contract to the Library of Congress, for distribution throughout the U.S. Also produces braille materials for schools, businesses, and other organizations.

Association for Education and Rehabilitation
of the Blind and Visually Impaired
206 N. Washington St., Ste. 320
Alexandria, VA 22314
(703) 548-1844
Formed in 1984 by the merger of the American Association of Workers for the Blind and the Association for Education of the Visually Handicapped, this association addresses the needs of professionals charged with providing services to people with visual impairments. Publishes *AER Report*, a bimonthly newsletter for professionals in the field.

Braille Institute of America, Inc.
741 N. Vermont Ave.
Los Angeles, CA 90029
(213) 663-1111
Produces textbooks, fiction, and general nonfiction including cookbooks and *Expectations* (annual), an anthology of children's fiction in braille, which is distributed free to blind children ages 6 through 13 worldwide.

Clovernook Printing House for the Blind
7000 Hamilton Ave.
Cincinnati, OH 45231
(513) 522-3860
Producer of braille books, magazines, catalogs, and other publications for national organizations, including the National Library Service, American Foundation for the Blind, Lions Clubs, and various U.S. government agencies.

Fliptrack One on One
Computer Training
2055 Army Trail Rd., Ste. 100
Addison, IL 60101

(708) 628-0500
Producer of audio format computer tutorials. Audio cassettes are accompanied by program-specific training disks.

Georgetown Center for Texts and Technology
Georgetown University
Washington, DC 20057
(202) 687-6096
The Center is currently working on a full catalog of resources for obtaining electronic texts. At present, a partial listing is available through LIST SERV@BROWNVM or via Bitnet: get PROJECTSETEXTS HUMANIST.

Jewish Guild for the Blind
15 W. 65th St.
New York, NY 10023
(212) 769-6200
Founded in 1914, this is a volunteer service agency for blind, visually impaired, and multihandicapped people of all ages, races, and creeds. Provides social services, rehabilitation, mobility and orientation training, medical services, group and recreational programs, etc. Operates In Touch Network, a 24-hour reading service for blind and visually impaired persons. Produces texts in both braille and audio format.

National Braille Association, Inc. (NBA)
Braille Book Bank
1290 University Ave.
Rochester, NY 14607
Produces college textbooks, general interest nonfiction, dictionaries, foreign language instructional materials, technical tables, and music. Printed catalogs available.

National Braille Press
88 Saint Stephen St.
Boston, MA 02115
(617) 266-6160
Independent publishers of texts of interest to blind and visually impaired readers. Most books are produced in a variety of accessible formats including audio cassette, braille, and machine-readable. Sponsors a children's Braille Book-of-the-Month Club.

National Library Service for the Blind and Physically Handicapped
1291 Taylor St. NW
Washington, DC 20542
(202) 287-5100
Produces reading materials of general interest in a variety of accessible formats including audio cassette, braille, flexible disc, and large print. The

NLS maintains a network of regional libraries through which qualified users may borrow books by mail.

Online Book Initiative (OBI)
1330 Beacon St.
Brookline, MA 02146
This project produces texts as well as maps and other graphics-based materials in electronic format.

Project Gutenberg
Illinois Benedictine College
5700 College Rd.
Lisle, IL 60532
Bitnet: HART@UIUCVMD
Internet: HART@VMD.CSO.UIUC.EDU
This project, spearheaded by Michael Hart at the University of Illinois, has produced a number of public domain texts in machine-readable format. Users may download these text files free of charge via modem. While the current collection is quite small, plans are underway to increase Project Gutenberg's holdings, with the goal of 10,000 texts online by the year 2000.

Random House AUDIO BOOKS
1-800-726-0600
Publishers of audio cassette versions of popular books in abridged format. Tapes are purchased directly from the company or in retail bookstores.

Recording for the Blind, Inc.
20 Rozsel Rd.,
Princeton, NJ 08540
1-800-221-4792
Producers of academic texts in recorded and electronic format. Like NLS, RFB maintains a series of cooperating libraries across the country through which members may borrow audio cassettes. The e-texts are purchased from RFB directly.

Volunteer Braillists, Inc.
5930 Old Sauk Rd.
Madison, WI 53705
Fiction and general nonfiction, including cookbooks, child care, children's literature. Free loan to residents of the United States; also available for purchase at 5 to 10 cents per page plus cost of binding.

Womyn's Braille Press, Inc.
P.O. Box 8475
Minneapolis, MN 55408
(612) 872-4352
Small firm producing unabridged versions of feminist texts in recorded,

braille, and machine-readable format. Members may also subscribe to a number of magazines and journals. Texts in accessible formats may be borrowed or purchased.

Associations: Learning Disabilities

Council for Learning Disabilities
P.O. Box 40303
Overland Park, KS 66204
(913) 492-8755
Founded in 1967, this organization of professionals in the field of learning disabilities conducts research and disseminates information, primarily in education. Publishes *Learning Disability Quarterly.*

Learning Disabilities Association of America (LDA)
4156 Library Rd.
Pittsburgh, PA 15234
(412) 341-1515
Founded in 1964, this association is geared primarily toward parents of children with learning disabilities and professionals in fields of service to learning-disabled students. Publishes *LDA Newsbriefs* (bimonthly) and *Learning Disabilities*, a semiannual journal.

National Center for Learning Disabilities
99 Park Ave., 6th fl.
New York, NY 10016
(212) 687-7211
Founded in 1977, the Center provides information to volunteer and professional groups working with the learning disabled. Conducts seminars on a variety of topics relating to learning disabilities. Publishes *Their World* (annual).

Orton Dyslexia Society
724 York Rd.
Baltimore, MD 21204
(301) 296-0232
Founded in 1949 and named for Dr. Samuel T. Orton, a pioneer in the field of learning disabilities. The Society conducts research; holds workshops for professionals in education, psychiatry, social work, and psychology; and serves as a major clearinghouse of information on learning disabilities. Publishes *Annals of Dyslexia* (annual) and *Perspectives on Dyslexia* (quarterly).

Appendix B

Products and Vendors

Part I: Products

An alphabetical listing of the producers and/or vendors of the adaptive devices listed below can be found in part II of this appendix. Please note however, that the list is not exhaustive.

Braille

A. Soft Braille Systems

Included here are the notetakers and refreshable braille displays discussed in chapter 3.

ALVA Braille Terminal
Humanware, Inc.
Computer braille display which features 43 or 83 eight-dot braille cells. Displays vital information, such as location of system cursor and special screen attributes. Special touch cursor allows fast and accurate cursor routing.

Braille 'n Speak
Blazie Engineering
Converts braille input to synthetic speech. Weighing less than one pound, the Braille 'n Speak is used as a talking notetaker, clock, calendar, and telephone directory. Connects to PC via RS232 serial port.

BrailleMate
Telesensory Systems, Inc.
Hand-held computer featuring a braille keyboard, one 8-dot braille cell, and a built-in speech synthesizer. Optional memory card extends storage capacity. Software includes word processing, calendar, and telephone directory.

KeyBraille
Humanware, Inc.
Provides braille output from IBM and compatibles on a refreshable display. Five braille cells devoted to display line information. Available in 25- or 45-cell options.

Navigator
TeleSensory Systems, Inc.
Braille output computer system gives easy access to IBM PCs and compatibles. Many different configurations available. Display strip available with 20, 40, or 80 cells.

B. Braille Translation Programs

Braille Talk
GW Micro
Braille translation software converts standard ASCII text to grade 1 or grade 2 braille. Available for Apple and IBM computers and compatibles.

Duxbury Braille Translator
Duxbury Systems, Inc.
Available for both Macintosh and IBM compatible computers, converts standard ASCII text into formatted grade 2 braille. Foreign languages, as well as Nemeth code translation tables available.

Hot Dots
Raised Dot Computing, Inc.
IBM-PC braille translation program features grade 2 braille translation and back-translation, print formatter, and speech interface. Documentation provided in print, audio, or floppy disk.

PC Braille
Arts Computer Products, Inc.
Translation program converts text files into grade 1, grade 2, or computer braille. IBM and IBM-compatible PCs only.

C. Braille Printers
Braille Blazer Personal Braille Printer
Blazie Engineering
Braille printer equipped with speech output for setting parameters. Built-in sound muffler. Works with all IBM and compatible PCs.

Braille BookMaker
Enabling Technologies Co.
Braille embosser available for IBM and compatibles or Macintosh computers.

Embosses approximately 80 characters per second, and features inter-pointed, i.e., two-sided, braille printing.

Braille 'n Print
Humanware, Inc.
Connects to a Perkins Brailler to produce braille and print copy of documents. A 22K memory allows file storage. Slimline version attaches directly to the bottom of a Perkins Brailler; MK2MB version intended for multiuse settings.

Braillo 90
American Thermoform Corp.
Personal braille printer features 90 character-per-second printing speed. Printing speed as well as pressure adjustable.

Index Advance
Index Classic
Humanware, Inc.
Small, quiet, braille embossers. The Classic produces 25 characters per second; the Index Advance embosses at a rate of 50 characters per second. Available for Apple, Macintosh, and IBM computers and compatibles.

Ohtsuki BT-5000
American Thermoform Corp.
Braille printer has three modes of operation: braille embossing, ink print, or a combination of braille and print. Manufactured by Technol Eight Corporation.

Versapoint
TeleSensory Systems, Inc.
Available for Apple Macintosh, and IBM computers, this braille printer offers bidirectional line printing at 40 characters per second. Thirty thousand character buffer frees host computer for other work once file has been sent to the printer.

Synthetic Speech Hardware and Software

Each of the speech-based adaptive devices discussed in chapter 4 is identified, along with some other popular screen-access products.

Accent Speech Synthesizer
Aicom Corp.
Various models, including Accent PC (full-length PC plug-in card), Accent MC (microchannel), and a stand-alone version, the Accent SA.

Artic Vision
Business Vision
Artic Technologies, Inc.
Artic Vision is a sophisticated screen-access system used with IBM and compatibles. Business Vision incorporates a talking calculator and special spreadsheet functions with the standard Artic Vision software. Artic's software is designed to run only with the company's own Synphonix series of internal speech cards.

ASAP (Automated Screen-Access Program)
MicroTalk
Synthetic speech screen-access system used with IBM and compatible computers. Supports a variety of internal and external synthesizers. MicroTalk maintains speech-friendly support electronic bulletin board.

DECTalk Synthesizer
Digital Equipment Corp.
External device with remarkable sound quality. One of DECTalk's most popular features is its use of nine different voices. It should be noted, however, that this synthesizer's response time is notoriously slow.

ECHO series synthesizers
Street Electronics Corp.
Variety of models, both internal and external, compatible with all PCs and Apple II series.

Echo II with Textalker and Textalker-GS
American Printing House for the Blind
Complete speech synthesis program for Apple computers. Hardware consists of Echo II synthesizer, interface, and external speaker with volume control.

Flipper
Omnichron
Used with IBM and compatible computers, this software supports a number of internal and external synthesizers. Reports indicate that Flipper helps compensate for DECTalk's sluggish response time so that institutions which already own one of these synthesizers may consider purchasing this software. One of the program's outstanding features is its ability to handle terminal emulation.

IBM Screen-Reader
IBM Educational Systems
Combination hardware/software screen-access system features programmable 18-key external keypad to navigate screen. External keypad can minimize confusion for novice users. Note that the system was originally

designed to work with the company's PS/2 line of computers and, while the software will run with earlier versions of the PC, this requires an additional interface card. Screen-Reader does not, generally, support internal synthesizers.

JAWS (Job Access with Speech)
Henter-Joyce, Inc.
Screen-reading program features dual cursor design, built-in macros, logical speech pad, and help mode.

MasterTouch
Humanware, Inc.
Screen-access system that combines software with external touch tablet which provides users with a tactile representation of the full video display. Foreign language capabilities including French, Spanish, and German.

Outspoken
Berkeley Systems, Inc. (BSI)
Synthetic speech screen-access system used with the Apple Macintosh. Note that the software takes advantage of the Mac's built-in speech synthesizer so no additional hardware is required with this system.

Synphonix
Artic Technologies, Inc.
A series of internal synthesizers designed for use with IBM and compatible systems including all ISA bus desktop configurations, the IBM microchannel architecture, and Toshiba laptops. Note that running screen-access software other than Artic Business Vision with a Synphonix synthesizer requires the use of Artic's Sonix text to speech program (Sonixtts).

VERT Plus
TeleSensory Systems, Inc. (TSI)
Screen-access software used with IBM and compatible computers. Supports a number of internal and external speech synthesizers including TSI's own products. Features include user-definable windows, recognition of video attributes, and bar-tracking.

Vocal-eyes
GW Micro
Speech-based screen-access software used with IBM and compatible systems. The product was specifically designed for use with the Sounding Board (distributed by GW Micro as well) but supports several other synthesizers, both internal and external. Features include good interuptability and full review mode as well as secondary cursor.

OCR Technologies

The reading machines and multipurpose scanners introduced in chapter 2 are presented here along with other popular OCR devices.

Arkenstone Reader
Arkenstone, Inc.
The Arkenstone employs Calera TrueScan recognition software and a front-end user interface, EasyScan, to provide users with a high quality, speech-friendly recognition system. Includes a TrueScan Recognition Card, Hewlett-Packard scanner, and software.

DocuRead Expert
Adhoc Reading Systems, Inc.
Optical character recognition device intended for use by print-impaired users. Friendly to standard synthetic speech, soft braille, and screen-enlarging access systems. Full package includes scanner, interface card, and recognition software.

Kurzweil Personal Reader (KPR)
Xerox Imaging Systems, Inc.
Portable reading system that converts text to high quality DecTalk speech. Options include flatbed and hand scanners. System can be used in stand-alone mode for immediate speech output or interfaced with an IBM or compatible via serial port. Includes talking calculator.

OsCaR
TeleSensory Systems, Inc.
Optical character recognition system uses Calera TrueScan-E Recognition software with Hewlett-Packard scanner. Menu-driven system is very user friendly, permitting independent use by visually impaired readers.

PC/Kurzweil Personal Reader
Xerox Imaging Systems, Inc.
Unlike the KPR, this system is not a stand-alone unit but must be interfaced with an IBM or compatible PC. The flatbed scanner converts printed documents quickly and accurately into ASCII text files for output in braille, large print, or via synthetic-speech screen-access hardware and software.

Reading Aids for Low Vision

Each of the hardware and software devices described in chapter 5 is included along with some other popular aids for low-vision readers.

Clear View
Humanware, Inc.
A 14-inch CCTV features windowing, underlining and overlining, contrast,

and intensity and brightness controls. Zoom lens allows numerous magnification settings.

Compu-Lenz
Able-Tech Connection
The fresnel lens doubles the size of characters on computer display. Glare filter eliminates background glare. Requiring no power source or wiring, the Compu-Lenz is also lightweight and durable.

DP-11 Plus Large Print Display Processor
TeleSensory Systems, Inc.
A hardware device that enlarges characters into solid, proportional characters. Magnification options from 2 to 16 times. Enlarges all ASCII characters but does not support graphics. Designed for use with special monitor and IBM and compatible PCs.

Fonts-on-the-Fly
LaserTools Corp.
A software package that supplies WordPerfect with supplementary printer drivers for a diversity of scalable typefaces. Useful in the preparation of large-print hard copy.

InLarge
Berkeley Systems, Inc.
Large print software for Macintosh computers. Magnifies anything on the screen, including graphics, by 2 to 16 times. Can magnify the entire screen or selected portions.

Large Print DOS (LP DOS)
Optelec USA, Inc.
Software-based screen-enlarging system. Uses standard system keyboard to invoke magnification options. Drawbacks include a tendency to conflict with running applications.

Vantage CCD
TeleSensory Systems, Inc.
This CCTV device includes a 14-inch monitor. Magnification ranges from 3 to 45 times original size. May be used as a stand-alone CCTV device or with VISTA VGA for split-screen video display magnification.

Viewpoint
Humanware, Inc.
This portable CCTV features a 14-inch monitor, which is detachable from the camera and electronics. Optional second monitor.

Vista
TeleSensory Systems, Inc.
Large print computer screen-access device for IBM PCs and compatibles.

Uses a three-button mouse to control magnification as well as manual or automatic cursor. Enlarges graphics and text up to 16 times.

Voyager CCD
TeleSensory Systems, Inc.
This closed circuit television enlargement device features a 12-inch monitor and magnification up to 45 times. Electronic line markers isolate individual lines from rest of text. Features X/Y platform, fluorescent light source, monitor, and camera.

Voyager XL CCD
TeleSensory Systems, Inc.
A 19-inch diagonal black and white monitor CCTV. Magnification ranges to 60 times, electronic line markers, fluorescent light source. Can be interfaced with a computer, or used as a stand-alone enlargement device.

ZoomText Plus
Telesensory Systems, Inc.
Unobtrusive screen-enlarging TSR for IBM and compatibles. Uses menustem invoked by unusual key combination unlikely to interfere with software applications.

Part II: Vendors

Able Tech Connection
P.O. Box 898
Westerville, OH 43081
(614) 899-9989

Ad Hoc Reading Systems
28 Brunswick Woods Dr.
East Brunswick, NJ 08816
(201) 254-7300

Aicom Corp.
1590 Oakland Rd.
San Jose, CA 95131
(408) 453-8251

American Thermoform Corp.
2311 Travers Ave.
City of Commerce, CA 90040
(213) 723-9021

Arkenstone, Inc.
1185 Bordeaux Dr., Ste. D
Sunnyvale, CA 94089
(408) 752-2200

Artic Technologies
55 Park St. #2
Troy, MI 48083
(313) 588-7370

Arts Computer Products, Inc.
121 Beach St., Ste. 400
Boston, MA 02111
1-800-343-0095

Berkeley Systems, Inc.
2095 Rose St.
Berkeley, CA 94709
(510) 540-5535

Blazie Engineering
3660 Mill Green Rd.
Street, MD 21154
(301) 879-4944

Boston Information and
Technology Corp.
52 Roland St.
Boston, MA 02129-1122
1-800-333-2481

Digital Equipment Corp.
30 Forbes Rd.
Northboro, MA 01532
(508) 351-5205

Duxbury Systems, Inc.
435 King St., P.O. Box 1504
Littleton, MA 01460
(508) 486-9766

Enabling Technologies Co.
3102 S.E. Jay St.
Stuart, FL 34997
(407) 283-4817

GW Micro
310 Racquet Dr.
Fort Wayne, IA 46825
(219) 483-3625

Henter-Joyce, Inc.
816-75 Avenue N
St. Petersburg, FL 33716
(813) 576-5658
1-800-336-5658

Humanware, Inc.
6245 King Rd.
Loomis, CA 95650
(916) 652-7253

IBM Special Needs Information
Referral Center
c/o IBM Educational Systems
P.O. Box 2150
Atlanta, GA 30301-2150

1-800-426-2133
1-800-284-9482 (TDD)

LaserTools Corp.
1250 45th St., Ste. 100
Emeryville, CA 94608
1-800-767-8004

MicroTalk
3375 Peterson
Louisville, KY 40206
(502) 897-2705
(502) 893-2269 (modem)

Omnichron
6881 Sherwick Dr.
Berkeley, CA 94705
(415) 540-6455

Optelec USA, Inc.
4 Lyberty Way
Westford, MA 01886
(508) 392-0707

Raised Dot Computing, Inc.
408 S. Baldwin St.
Madison, WI 53703
(608) 257-9595

Street Electronics Corp.
6420 Via Real
Carpinteria, CA 93013
(805) 684-45493

Telesensory Systems, Inc.
455 N. Bernardo Ave.
Mountainview, CA 94039-7455
(415) 960-0920

Xerox Imaging Systems, Inc.
Centennial Dr.
Peabody, MA 01960
(508) 977-2000
1-800-343-0311

Appendix C

Resources for Locating Texts in Accessible Formats

APH-CARL
Online catalog of American Printing House for the Blind. Included are braille, recorded, and large print accessible texts.

Audio Cassette Finder: A Subject Guide to Literature Recorded on Audio Cassettes
1st ed. (1986)
(formerly *Index to Educational Audiotapes*)
Albuquerque, N.M.: National Information Center for Educational Media, 1986-

BLND
Library of Congress. National Library Service for the Blind and Physically Handicapped
The online version of the National Library Service Union Catalog, BLND lists over 120,000 items in braille and recorded format. Included are listings of recorded or braille items produced by the NLS itself, or by a number of other publishers of accessible format texts. Available to subscribers of BRS databases, pending approval by NLS.

Braille Book Review
Library of Congress. National Library Service for the Blind and Physically Handicapped (bimonthly)
Available in both print and braille editions, this bimonthly offers annotated reviews and notices of new braille books, as well as occasional and feature stories. An annual author/title index, issued separately, offers access to the

year's output of the National Library Service of books in braille and other accessible formats.

Braille Books
Library of Congress. National Library Service for the Blind and Physically Handicapped (annual)
Lists and briefly describes books published during the year by the National Library Service and other braille publishers. Includes author/title index. Available in braille and large print editions.

Cassette Books
Washington, D.C.: Library of Congress. National Library Service for the Blind and Physically Handicapped
Biennial, 1977/78–1979/80. Annual, 1981–
Annual listing of books on tape produced by or available from the National Library Service.

The Central Catalog: American Printing House for the Blind
Louisville, Ky. : American Printing House for the Blind (annual)
Contains listings of braille, recorded, and large print materials available from the American Printing House for the Blind. Includes both volunteer and commercially produced materials intended primarily for students.

The Complete Directory of Large Print Books and Serials
New York: R. R. Bowker, 1988–
Formerly *Large Type Books in Print*
Subject, author, and title indexes to the listings of over fifty large print publishers.

Directory of Portable Databases
Vol. 1, no. 1 (Jan. 1990)–
New York: Cuadra/Elsevier, 1990–
Annual compendium of CD-ROM and other database products. Includes CD-ROM, diskette, and magnetic tape products. Subject index and master index that identifies corresponding online databases and information sources.

E-kit
Princeton, N.J.: Recording for the Blind, Inc.
This series of machine-readable text files is provided free of charge to all RFB members. Included is a list of the agency's current e-text holdings and their prices, an explanation of how to purchase these materials, and an order form.

Foreign Language Books—Libros en Español
Washington, D.C.: The Library of Congress, National Library Service for the Blind and Physically Handicapped, 1984–

Music & Musicians: Large-Print Scores and Books Catalog
Washington, D.C.: Library of Congress. Division for the Blind and Physically Handicapped

Recording for the Blind: Catalog of Tape-Recorded Books
New York: Recording for the Blind, Inc., 1971/72–
Catalog of spoken word recordings. Kept up-to-date with supplements. RFB productions are also listed in BLND, the database of NLS.

Talking Book Topics
Library of Congress. National Library Service for the Blind and Physically Handicapped
This magazine is published bimonthly by the NLS on audio cassette, flexible disc, and in large print, and is designed to serve as an ongoing supplement to the library's main catalog of holdings.

Vision Resource List
Watertown, Mass.: Vision Foundation, Inc., 1988–
Lists large type reading materials produced by the Vision Foundation.

Words on Cassette
New York: R. R. Bowker Co., c1992–
Formed by merger of *Words on Tape* and *On Cassette*
Commercially produced unabridged spoken word recordings in print.

Appendix D

Selected Accessible- Format Reference Sources

Selected Audio Format Reference Sources

Not surprisingly, few major reference works have been produced in re-corded format. It takes but one encyclopedia and one dictionary to illustrate the unwieldiness of reference works on cassette or other recorded media: the *World Book Encyclopedia* comprises 219 tapes, recorded at half the speed of commercial audio cassettes, and the *"Concise" Heritage Dictionary* is anything but concise, requiring 56 cassettes.

The Concise Heritage Dictionary—Recorded Ed.
Boston: Houghton Mifflin, c1976
56 sound cassettes

The World Book Encyclopedia—Recorded Ed.
Louisville, Ky.: American Printing House for the Blind, 1981
219 sound cassettes (19 v.)
Each volume has its own index and contains the contents of the cassette in braille. Instructions for use are inserted between the braille contents and index. The recorded edition was produced from the 1980 edition of *World Book Encyclopedia*. Updated by annual yearbooks.

Selected Large Print Reference Works

Castillo and Bond. *University of Chicago Spanish Dictionary: A New Concise Spanish-English & English-Spanish Dictionary of Words and Phrases Basic to the Written & Spoken Language of Today.* 8 vols. Large type ed. 1,740p. 11 by 12 1/2, 18-point type. Reprint of 1948 edition. American Printing House for the Blind

Consumer Reports Buying Guide Issue. Annual. Large type ed. Approx. 400p. Grey Castle

Coulson, Jessie, ed. *The Little Oxford Dictionary of Current English.* Large type ed. 5 1/2 by 8 3/4, 16-pt. type. Ulverscroft

Dutch, R. *Roget's Thesaurus of English Words & Phrases*, 12 vols. New, rev large type ed. 2,672p. 11 by 12 1/2, 18-point type. Reprint of 1962 edition. American Printing House for the Blind

Follet Vest-Pocket Dictionary: French English, English French. Compiled by R. Switzer. 2 vols. Large type ed. 11 by 12 1/2, 18-point type. Reprint of 1962 edition. American Printing House for the Blind

Hammond Large Type World Atlas. Large type ed. (illus). 9 3/8 by 12 1/4, 13- to 36-point type. 1984. Hammond, Inc. (Distributed by G. K. Hall)

ISIS Large Print English Dictionary. Large type ed. (Mainstream Series). 216p. 6 by 9, 16-point type. ABC-CLIO

ISIS Large Print Medical Dictionary. Large type ed. (Mainstream Series). 216p. 6 by 9, 16-point type. 1985. ABC-CLIO

ISIS Large Print Thesaurus. Large type ed. (Mainstream Series). 864p. 6 by 9. 16-point type. 1985. ABC-CLIO

Kribbs, Jayne K. *Annotated Bibliography of American Literary Periodicals, 1741-1850.* Large type ed. 6 by 9, 16-point type. 1977. G. K. Hall

The Little Oxford Dictionary. 6th Large type ed. 5 1/2 by 8 3/4. 16-point type. 1987. Ulverscroft

Scott, Foresman Beginning Dictionary. Edited by Thorndike and Barnhart. 5 vols. Large type edition. 1,500p. 11 by 12 1/2, 16-point type. 1982. Reprint of 1979 edition, American Printing House for the Blind

Webster's Intermediate Dictionary, 14 vols. Large type ed. 3,876p. 11 by 12 1/2. 16 - to 18-point type. American Printing House for the Blind

Webster's New World Dictionary of the American Language: Second College Edition. Edited by David B. Guralnik. 24 vols. Large type ed. 11 by 12 1/2, 18-point type.

Weisse, Fran A., and Mimi Winer. *Coping with Sight Loss: The Vision Resource Book.* Large type ed. 219p. 8 1/2 by 11, 20-point type. 1980. Vision Foundation

Selected Machine-Readable Reference Works

CompuBIBLE
Vendor: Nassco
Format: 3 1/2- or 5 1/4-inch disk
System requirements: IBM PC or compatible; two floppy drives or hard
  disk; 384 K memory
Contains the complete text of *American Standard Version, King James Version,
New International Version, New King James Version,* and *Revised Standard
Version.* Each version includes both the Old and New Testament. Also
includes Strong's *Concordance.* Software enables the user to view any four
translations simultaneously.

Directories in Print
Vendor: Gale Research, Inc.
Format: 3 1/2- or 5 1/4-inch diskette
System requirements: IBM PC, PS/2, or compatible; floppy drive; hard
  disk; 640K memory; monochrome or color monitor
Contains references to about 18,500 directories published in the United
States and abroad. Covers all subject areas. For each directory, includes
name and address of publisher, number of listings, content description,
arrangement of entries, frequency, and online availability.

The Electronic Encyclopedia/Grolier
CD-ROM version
Vendor: Grolier Electronic Publishing, Inc.
System requirements: IBM PC, PS/2, or compatible; 512K of memory;
  VGA card and monitor; CD-ROM drive
Contains full-text images of the 21-volume *Academic American Encyclopedia,*
1990 edition. Includes more than 33,000 articles on a wide variety of
subjects. Entries are indexed by subject and include tables, fact boxes,
bibliographies, and cross-references. Full-text images appear in the original
volumes and include all photographs and other illustrations. Corresponds
to the *Academic American Encyclopedia* online database.

Encyclopedia of Associations
Vendor: Gale Research, Inc.
Format: 3 1/2- or 5 /4-inch diskette
System requirements: same as above
Contains descriptions of 22,000 U.S. national associations; 47,000 U.S.
associations with local, state, or regional scope or membership; and 10,000
international and national associations with interests outside the U.S. Up-
dated twice annually.

Hyper-ABLEDATA on diskette
Vendor: Trace Center
Format: 3 1/2- or 5 1/4-inch diskette
System requirements: Apple Macintosh Plus, SE, or II Series
Contains more than 16,000 descriptions, including illustrations and sound samples, of products and equipment useful to persons with disabilities. Covers personal care, therapeutic, sensory, educational, vocational, transportation, and other types of technical items. Information provided for each product includes generic name, brand name (i.e., trade name and/or model number), manufacturer's name, address, telephone. Corresponds in part to the ABLEDATA database (available online through BRS).

McGraw-Hill CD-ROM Science and Technical Reference Set
Vendor: McGraw-Hill Publishing Co.
System requirements: IBM PC or compatible; two 5 1/4-inch floppy drives; 640K memory; monochrome or color monitor (VGA monitor required to display images); CD-ROM drive
Part I: Contains complete text of the *McGraw Hill Concise Encyclopedia of Science & Technology* (2d ed.). Over 7,000 articles covering 77 major scientific and technological subject areas. Also includes all photographs and illustrations. Corresponds to the *McGraw-Hill Concise Encyclopedia of Science and Technology* online database.
Part II: *McGraw Hill Dictionary of Scientific and Technical Terms*. Contains 100,100 scientific and technical terms with 117,500 definitions. Corresponds to *McGraw Hill Dictionary of Scientific and Technical Terms* (4th ed.).

Microsoft Bookshelf
Vendor: Microsoft Corp.
System requirements: IBM PC, PS/2 or compatible computer; 640K memory; CD-ROM drive
Contains 10 popular reference works:
1987 World Almanac and Book of Facts; *American Heritage Dictionary*; *Bartlett's Familiar Quotations*; *Business Information Sources*; *Chicago Manual of Style*; *Forms and Letters*; *Houghton Mifflin Spelling Verifier and Corrector*; *Houghton Mifflin Usage Alert*; *Roget's II: Electronic Thesaurus*; *U.S. Zip Code Directory*.

World Atlas
Vendor: The Software Toolworks, Inc.
Format: 3 1/2- or 5 1/4-inch diskette
System requirements: IBM PC or compatible; floppy drive; hard disk with 5 MB free; 640K memory; EGA or VGA card and monitor; mouse
Contains over 235 world, country, regional, topographic, and other maps. For each country, also includes information and statistics in 45 areas, covering geography, people, government, economy, and communications. Descriptive information can be displayed on the screen with associated maps.

Bibliography

Andersson, Torsten. "Microfiche as a Reading Aid for Partially Sighted Students." *Journal of Visual Impairment and Blindness* 74 (May 1980): 193–96.

Anthony, Carolyn. "More Eyes on Large Print: With New Players in the Field, Older and Younger Readers Are Getting a Wider Choice of Titles and Faster Delivery of Bestsellers." *Publishers Weekly* 238 (Jan. 25, 1991): 18–23.

Barraga, Natalie C. "Utilization of Low Vision in Adults Who Are Severely Visually Handicapped." *New Outlook for the Blind* 70 (May 1976): 177–81.

Basch, Reva. "Books On-line: Visions, Plans and Perspectives for Electronic Texts." *Online* 15 (July 1991): 13–23.

Baskin, Barbara H., and Karen H. Harris. *The Mainstreamed Library: Issues, Ideas, Innovations.* Chicago: American Library Assn., 1982.

Bliss, Barbara. "Dyslexics as Library Users." *Library Trends* 35 (Fall 1986): 293–302.

Bliss, James C., and Mary W. Moore. "The Optacon Reading System." In *The Mainstreamed Library: Issues, Ideas, Innovations,* 107.

Braille Instruction and Writing Equipment. Reference Circular no. 86-3. Washington, D.C.: Library of Congress. National Library Service for the Blind and Physically Handicapped, March 1986.

Boyd, Lawrence H., Wesley L. Boyd, and Gregg. C. Vanderheiden. "The Graphical User Interface: Crisis, Danger and Opportunity." *Journal of Visual Impairment and Blindness* 84 (Dec. 1990): 496–502.

Carroll, Thomas J., and others. *Standards for Production of Reading Materials for the Blind and Visually Handicapped.* New York: National Accreditation Council for Agencies Serving Blind and Visually Handicapped, Sept. 1970 (ERIC Document Reproduction Service, ED 056 709).

Connor, Aikin. "A Comparison of Traditional Large Type and Microfiche as Reading Modes for Low Vision Students." *Journal of Micrographics* 14 (Nov. 1981): 32–38.

Cooper, Franklin S. "Research on Reading Machines for the Blind." In *Blindness: Modern Approaches to the Unseen Environment.* Ed. Paul A. Zahl, 512–43. Princeton, N.J.: Princeton University Press, 1950.

Corn, A. "Access to Print for Students with Low Vision." *Journal of Visual Impairment and Blindness* 83 (Spring 1989): 340–49.

Currid, Cheryl. "Corporate Reflections on the PC's 10th Birthday," *PC Week* 8 (Aug. 5, 1991): 64.

De Witt, J. C., and others. "Guide to Selecting Large Print/Enhanced Image Computer Access Hardware/Software for Persons with Low Vision." *Journal of Visual Impairment and Blindness* 82 (Dec. 1988): 432–42.

Directory of Services for Blind and Visually Impaired Persons in the United States. 23d ed. New York: American Foundation for the Blind, 1988.

Dixon, Judith M., and Jane B. Mandalbaum. "Reading through Technology: Evolving Methods and Opportunities for Print-Handicapped Individuals." *Journal of Visual Impairment and Blindness* 84 (Dec. 1990): 493–96.

Dixon, Lana S. "The Visually Impaired and the Academic Library." *College & Research Libraries News* 51 (July/Aug. 1990): 637–38.

Dreyfus, John. "The Invention of Spectacles and the Advent of Printing." *The Library.* 6th Ser. 10, no. 2 (June 1988): 93–106.

Facciarossa, Laurie. RFB public information officer. Telephone interview with Dawn M. Suvino, New York, January 27, 1992.

FACTS. Washington D.C.: Library of Congress, National Library Service for the Blind and Physically Handicapped, January 1991.

Faye, Eleanor E. *Clinical Low Vision.* Boston: Little, Brown, 1976.

Fitzpatrick, Vicki. "The Sole Source: The Library of Congress National Library Service for the Blind and Physically Handicapped." *Health Libraries Review* 7 (1990): 73–85.

Gartner, John N. "Large Type Reading Materials for the Visually Handicapped." *New Outlook for the Blind* 62 (October 1968): 233–39.

Goldberg, A. M., and others. "An Evaluation of Braille Translation Programs." *Journal of Visual Impairment and Blindness* 81 (Dec. 1987): 193, 195–96.

Guidelines for the Production of Materials in Large Type. New York: National Society for the Prevention of Blindness, 1965.

Guidelines for the Production of Reading Materials for the Blind and Visually Handicapped. New York: National Accreditation Council for Agencies Serving the Blind and Visually Handicapped, 1970.

Harris, Elizabeth M. "Inventing Printing for the Blind." *Printing History* 8 (1986): 15–25.

"High Quality Service Meets Special Needs." *Library of Congress Informational Bulletin* 50 (March 25, 1991): 97–104.

Hooker, Fran. "Computerized Braille: The Boulder Story." *Wilson Library Bulletin* 59 (April 1985): 527–30.

Irwin, Robert B. *Classes for the Conservation of Vision.* Manuscript. 1916.

Jahoda, Gerald, and Elizabeth A. Johnson. "The Use of the Kurzweil Reading Machine in Academic Libraries." *Journal of Academic Librarianship* (May 1987): 99–101.

Kazlauskas, Diane W., Sharon T. Weaver, and William R. Jones. "Kurzweil Reading Machine: A Study of Usage Patterns." *Journal of Academic Librarianship* (Jan. 1987): 356–58.

Kerscher, George. Telephone interview with Dawn M. Suvino, New York, February 13, 1992.

Large Print Book Project: A Report. New York: New York Public Library, 1969.

Lazzaro, Joseph J. "Hearing Graphics for the First Time." *Screen Reader Newsletter* 3 (Jan. 1992): 24–25.

Leventhal, J. AFB National Technology Center. Personal interview with Dawn M. Suvino, New York, January 22, 1992.

Leventhal, J., and others. "A Guide to Paperless Braille Devices." *Journal of Visual Impairment and Blindness* 82 (Sept. 1988): 290–96.

Library Service for Persons with Disabilities: SPEC Kit 176. Washington, D.C.: Systems and Procedures Exchange Center, OMS, Association of College and Research Libraries, July/Aug. 1991.

Luxton, Karen. Director, Computer Center for the Visually Impaired, Baruch College, City University of New York. Personal interview with Tom McNulty, January 31, 1992.

Mack, Catherine. "The Impact of Technology on Braille Literacy." *Journal of Visual Impairment and Blindness* 83 (June 1989): 314.

Massis, Bruce E. Librarian, Jewish Guild for the Blind. Telephone interview with Tom McNulty, April 26, 1992.

———. *The International Guide to Publishers and Distributors of Large Print IFLA Professional Reports,* no. 4. The Hague: International Federal of Library Associations, 1985. (ERIC Document Reproduction Service, ED 264 862).

Melton, Louise. "Mister Impossible: Ray Kurzweil." *Computers & Electronics* 22 (July 1984): 40–49.

Meyers, Andrea, and Elliot Schreier. "An Evaluation of Speech Access Programs." *Journal of Visual Impairment and Blindness* 84 (Jan. 1990): 26–38.

Mosakowski, Susan. Director of talking book recording studio, New York Regional Library for the Blind. Personal interview with Dawn M. Suvino, New York, January 27, 1992.

Neville, Ann, and John Kupersmith, "Online Access for Visually Impaired Students." *Database* 14 (Dec. 1991): 102–5.

Ong, Walter. *Orality and Literacy: The Technologizing of the Word.* New York: Methuen, 1982.

Palmer, Judith Lee. "Large-Print Books: Public Library Services to Older Adults." *Educational Gerontology* 14 (1988): 211–20.

Projects and Experiments. Washington, D.C.: Library of Congress, National Library Service for the Blind and Physically Handicapped, Summer 1990.

Reading Materials in Large Type. Reference Circular no. 87-4, Washington, D.C.: Library of Congress. National Library Service, July 1987.

Redmond, Linda, "Large Print Books and Magazines." In *Encyclopedia of Library and Information Science.* vol. 37, supp. 2. Executive editor, Allen Kent. New York: Marcel Dekker.

Rosen, Leslie. "Enabling Blind and Visually Impaired Library Users: In-Magic and Adaptive Technologies." *Library Hi Tech* 9 (1991): 55–61.

Roth, Joel A. "Low-Vision Readers." *Talking Book Topics* 31 (Sept. 1965): 140.

Schwerdtfeger, Richard S. "Making the GUI Talk." *Byte* 16 (Dec. 1991): 118.

Sorsby, Arnold. "Blindness in the World Today." *WHO Chronicle* 21 (Sept. 1967): 369–73.

Spungin, Susan J. *Braille Literacy: Issues for Blind Persons, Families, Professionals, and Producers of Braille.* New York: American Foundation for the Blind, n.d.

Stocker, Claudell S. Head, Braille Development Division, National Library Service for the Blind, Library of Congress. "Volunteer Braille Transcribing in the United States." Manuscript, n.d.

That All May Read: Library Service for the Blind and Physically Handicapped. Washington, D.C.: Library of Congress, National Library Service for the Blind and Physically Handicapped, 1983.

Vanderplas, James M., and Jean H. Vanderplas. "Some Factors Affecting Legibility of Printed Materials for Older Adults." *Perceptual and Motor Skills* 50 (June 1980): 923–32.

Velleman, Ruth A. *Meeting the Needs of People with Disabilities: A Guide for Librarians, Educators, and Other Service Professionals.* Phoenix, Ariz.: Oryx, 1990.

Volunteers Who Produce Books: Braille, Tape, Large Print. Washington, D.C.: Library of Congress. National Library Service for the Blind and Physically Handicapped, 1988.

Votta, Myrna. New York Association for the Blind. Personal interview with Dawn M. Suvino, New York, March 6, 1992.

Wilkinson, John. Literary Braille Adviser, National Library Service for the Blind and Physically Handicapped. Telephone interview with Tom McNulty, March 3, 1992.

Wolfe, Diane. New York Public Library for the Blind and Physically Handicapped. Personal interview with Dawn M. Suvino, New York, January 27, 1992.

———. Telephone interview with Tom McNulty, March 25, 1992.

World Braille Usage. Paris: UNESCO; Washington, D.C.: Library of Congress, National Library Service for the Blind and Physically Handicapped, 1990.

Zahl, Paul E., ed. *Blindness: Modern Approaches to the the Unseen Environment.* Princeton, N.J.: Princeton Univ. Pr., 1950.

Index

Dawn M. Suvino, Technology Instructor at the Westchester Lighthouse for the Blind, has ten years' experience as a freelance consultant and classroom instructor in computer applications. She holds a master's degree in French literature from New York University and is currently a doctoral candidate in the Department of Linguistics, University of Pennsylvania.

Tom McNulty, a paraprofessional reference librarian at New York University's Bobst Library, serves as library liaison to the University's Center for Students with Disabilities. He holds a master's degree in fine arts from New York University and is currently pursuing a master's of library science degree at Queens College, City University of New York.